Fetal Alcohol Disorders

Diseases and Disorders

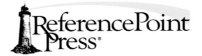

ReferencePoint
Press®

San Diego, CA

Other books in the Compact Research Diseases and Disorders set:

ADHD
Alzheimer's Disease
Anorexia
Anxiety Disorders
Asthma
Autism
Bipolar Disorders
Brain Tumors
Diabetes
Down Syndrome
Drug Addiction
Epilepsy
Food-Borne Illnesses
Genetic Disorders
Hepatitis
Herpes
HPV
Influenza
Learning Disabilities
Leukemia
Meningitis
Mood Disorders
Obsessive-Compulsive Disorder
Personality Disorders
Phobias
Post-Traumatic Stress Disorder
Schizophrenia
Self-Injury Disorder
Sexually Transmitted Diseases
Sleep Disorders

*For a complete list of titles please visit www.referencepointpress.com.

Fetal Alcohol Disorders

Sandra Alters

Diseases and Disorders

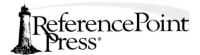

ReferencePoint Press®

San Diego, CA

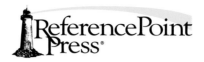

© 2012 ReferencePoint Press, Inc.
Printed in the United States

For more information, contact:
ReferencePoint Press, Inc.
PO Box 27779
San Diego, CA 92198
www.ReferencePointPress.com

Picture credits:
Cover: Dreamstime and iStockphoto.com
Maury Aaseng: 34–36, 48–49, 62–64, 78–79
AP Images: 17
Landov: 11

LIBRARY OF CONGRESS CATALOGING-IN-PUBLICATION DATA

Alters, Sandra.
  Fetal alcohol disorders / by Sandra M. Alters.
     p. cm. — (Compact research series)
  Includes bibliographical references and index.
  ISBN-13: 978-1-60152-159-0 (hardback)
  ISBN-10: 1-60152-159-6 (hardback)
   1. Fetal alcohol syndrome. 2. Children of prenatal alcohol abuse. 3. Alcoholism in pregnancy.
I. Title.
  RG629.F45.A48   2011
  618.3'26861—dc22

                                                    2010047305

Contents

Foreword

Foreword

66**Where is the knowledge we have lost in information?**99

—T.S. Eliot, "The Rock."

As modern civilization continues to evolve, its ability to create, store, distribute, and access information expands exponentially. The explosion of information from all media continues to increase at a phenomenal rate. By 2020 some experts predict the worldwide information base will double every 73 days. While access to diverse sources of information and perspectives is paramount to any democratic society, information alone cannot help people gain knowledge and understanding. Information must be organized and presented clearly and succinctly in order to be understood. The challenge in the digital age becomes not the creation of information, but how best to sort, organize, enhance, and present information.

ReferencePoint Press developed the *Compact Research* series with this challenge of the information age in mind. More than any other subject area today, researching current issues can yield vast, diverse, and unqualified information that can be intimidating and overwhelming for even the most advanced and motivated researcher. The *Compact Research* series offers a compact, relevant, intelligent, and conveniently organized collection of information covering a variety of current topics ranging from illegal immigration and deforestation to diseases such as anorexia and meningitis.

The series focuses on three types of information: objective single-author narratives, opinion-based primary source quotations, and facts and statistics. The clearly written objective narratives provide context and reliable background information. Primary source quotes are carefully selected and cited, exposing the reader to differing points of view. And facts and statistics sections aid the reader in evaluating perspectives. Presenting these key types of information creates a richer, more balanced learning experience.

For better understanding and convenience, the series enhances information by organizing it into narrower topics and adding design features that make it easy for a reader to identify desired content. For example, in *Compact Research: Illegal Immigration*, a chapter covering the economic impact of illegal immigration has an objective narrative explaining the various ways the economy is impacted, a balanced section of numerous primary source quotes on the topic, followed by facts and full-color illustrations to encourage evaluation of contrasting perspectives.

The ancient Roman philosopher Lucius Annaeus Seneca wrote, "It is quality rather than quantity that matters." More than just a collection of content, the *Compact Research* series is simply committed to creating, finding, organizing, and presenting the most relevant and appropriate amount of information on a current topic in a user-friendly style that invites, intrigues, and fosters understanding.

Fetal Alcohol Disorders at a Glance

A Spectrum of Disorders

Fetal alcohol disorders—more technically known as fetal alcohol spectrum disorders—are a range of conditions caused by exposure to alcohol in the womb.

Causes

Alcohol consumption during pregnancy can result in fetal alcohol disorders.

Effects

Exposure to alcohol in the womb can damage the brain, heart, and other organs during development. This damage can lead to physiological challenges, intellectual deficits, behavioral problems, and learning difficulties.

Prevalence

No one knows exactly how many people in the United States or worldwide are living with fetal alcohol disorders. Estimates are that these disorders affect about 40,000 newborns each year in the United States, or almost 1 percent of newborns annually.

Diagnosis

Diagnosing a fetal alcohol disorder can be difficult and usually requires a team of medical professionals.

Prevention

Fetal alcohol disorders are 100 percent preventable if women abstain from drinking alcohol when they are pregnant.

Early Intervention

A variety of steps can be taken to help a child with a fetal alcohol disorder succeed and increase well-being in both the classroom and at home.

Difficulties for Adults

Most adults with fetal alcohol disorders cannot live on their own because of their disabilities, which can easily compromise their safety or the safety of others.

Overview

❝There is no known amount of alcohol use that is safe during pregnancy. There is no known time during pregnancy when alcohol use is safe.❞

—Centers for Disease Control and Prevention.

❝Millions of children and adults worldwide are struggling with lost intellectual potential caused by prenatal alcohol, and most will never be diagnosed.❞

—Bonnie Buxton, adoptive mother of a girl with fetal alcohol syndrome.

Although it is hard for her to read and write, Katia Demchuk is not embarrassed. On the contrary, the teenager is determined to talk about her challenges in order to help others with similar problems. When she was a fourth grader she did just that, traveling from her hometown in Brunswick, Ohio, to Capitol Hill to tell lawmakers what life is like with fetal alcohol syndrome, or FAS. Demchuk wants to raise the public's awareness of her condition and promote the understanding that drinking alcohol during pregnancy poses serious dangers to the fetus.

What Are Fetal Alcohol Disorders?

Fetal alcohol disorders are a spectrum of conditions that result from the effects of alcohol on an embryo or fetus during pregnancy. This array of conditions is more technically referred to as fetal alcohol spectrum disorders, or FASD. Fetal alcohol syndrome (FAS) is the most severe of these disorders. Other less severe FASDs include partial fetal alcohol syndrome, alcohol-

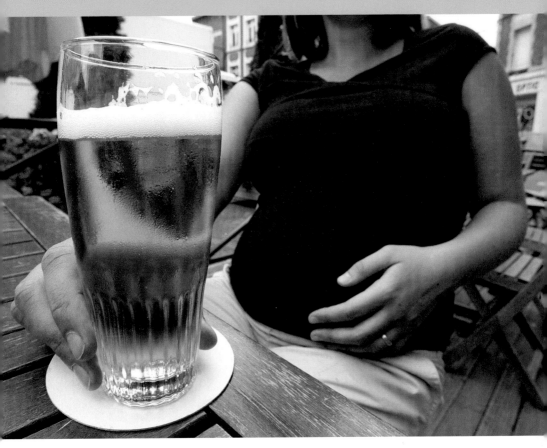

Drinking beer, wine, or liquor during pregnancy poses serious dangers to the fetus. Abnormal growth and mental retardation are among possible consequences of alcohol consumption during pregnancy.

related neurodevelopmental disorder, and alcohol-related birth defects.

Exposure to alcohol in the womb results in varying effects among individuals, which is one reason why FASD is a continuum of conditions. The type and severity of a fetal alcohol disorder also depends on the prebirth alcohol exposure. The amount and timing of drinking by a pregnant woman is an important factor in the type and severity of effects on her embryo or fetus, but no exact relationship has been determined. Nevertheless, there is no safe level of alcohol consumption during pregnancy.

Previously Noted but Not Named

References to alcohol-related birth defects can be found in the writings of Aristotle and in the Bible. In the eighteenth century, English physicians described the problems experienced by children who were born to alcoholic mothers. Nevertheless, until 1973 fetal alcohol syndrome had no formal medical description and no name. The phrase was coined by pediatrician David Smith and his research associate Kenneth Lyons Jones, at the time working at the University of Washington School of Medicine in Seattle.

> " Fetal alcohol disorders are a spectrum of conditions that result from the effects of alcohol on an embryo or fetus during pregnancy. "

The physicians were experts in dysmorphology—interpreting patterns of physical characteristics to diagnose disorders. Because of his expertise, Smith was called to the Harborview Medical Center—part of the University of Washington—to examine 8 children born of alcoholic mothers. He and his associate Jones noticed that 4 of the 8 children had these same characteristics: a small head circumference, mental deficiencies, and growth deficiencies. In addition, the pair determined that these patterns existed in 2 children described in their research files who were also born of alcoholic mothers.

Within days, the medical researchers found an additional two children from other hospitals with the same abnormalities who were born of alcoholic mothers. Smith and Jones worked with clinical psychologist Ann Streissguth to test the children. They also worked with pediatrician Christy Ulleland, who had recently recognized and described the abnormalities in children at Harborview. Jones, Smith, Ulleland, and Streissguth wrote up their findings, which were published in the June 9, 1973, issue of the esteemed British medical journal the *Lancet*. In a second *Lancet* article published five months later, Smith and Jones first used the diagnostic phrase "fetal alcohol syndrome." The term is still in use today.

Sorting Out the Problem

According to the National Organization on Fetal Alcohol Syndrome, most children with a fetal alcohol spectrum disorder are either undiagnosed or misdiagnosed. These children may have brain damage and exhibit learning or behavioral difficulties, but these difficulties may not point directly to a fetal alcohol disorder. Michael Dorris, in his award-winning book *The Broken Cord*, describes his years of trying to understand what was wrong with his adopted son, Adam, who was later diagnosed with FAS:

> My recognition that Adam had a problem more serious than a "slow start" came in bits and pieces over the course of many years. In retrospect, the signs were all there, but at the time I stored in a file of nagging worry the poor hearing, the convulsions, the hundreds of repetitions of even the most basic instructions, the abbreviated attention span, the many minor, dismissable incidents, mistakes, and shortfalls. Finally, the accumulation became so numerous, so insistent, that anxiety spilled into my every thought. Yet even then, my capacity for rationalization proved almost limitless.[1]

As Adam's father described, children with a fetal alcohol disorder may have convulsions, a short attention span, and difficulty hearing. Other problems may include hyperactivity, the inability to focus on or complete tasks, disruptiveness, poor social skills, impulsivity, and a disregard for authority. However, *many* children have some or all of these problems and do not have a fetal alcohol disorder. Thus, students with behavioral and/or learning disabilities must undergo psychological and educational testing to try to determine the root cause of their problems.

Diagnosis of Fetal Alcohol Disorders

Diagnosis usually requires a team of medical professionals that may include physicians, psychiatrists, geneticists, psychologists, and speech pathologists. The most severe of these disorders, fetal alcohol syndrome, is the easiest to diagnose because the signs are more obvious. Along with having many of the challenges already mentioned, the FAS child has patterns of problems in three areas that are recognizable to physicians: slowed growth, abnormal facial features, and central nervous system dysfunction. Fetal alcohol syndrome can be diagnosed with or without a confirmed pattern of excessive drinking by the mother.

Children who do not have all the characteristics of FAS may be diagnosed with partial FAS, alcohol-related neurodevelopmental disorder, or alcohol-related birth defects. These diagnoses are generally not made without a confirmed pattern of excessive drinking by the mother. For instance, a child with known maternal alcohol use during pregnancy but without the abnormal facial features of FAS may be diagnosed with alcohol-related neurodevelopmental disorder. As its name suggests, this disorder includes the neurological and developmental abnormalities of an FASD, such as small head size at birth and impaired fine and gross motor skills. In addition, a child with this disorder may have behavioral or cognitive issues.

> According to the National Organization on Fetal Alcohol Syndrome, most children with a fetal alcohol spectrum disorder are either undiagnosed or misdiagnosed.

A child with a diagnosis of alcohol-related birth defects may have one or more birth defects related to the mother's known drinking during pregnancy. These birth defects include malformations and abnormal development of the heart, bones, or kidneys. They may also affect vision and hearing.

The Prevalence of Fetal Alcohol Disorders

According to researchers at the National Institutes of Health, FASD affects about 40,000 newborns each year, which is almost 1 percent of newborns annually—about 10 out of every 1,000. FASD affects more infants each year than muscular dystrophy (a disorder of the muscles), spina bifida (incomplete closure of the vertebrae around the spinal cord), and Down syndrome (a genetic disorder) combined. It is not known how many people in the United States or worldwide are living with a fetal alcohol disorder.

What Is the Cause of Fetal Alcohol Disorders?

When a woman is pregnant, the organism developing within her relies on her body for oxygen and nourishment. These substances are brought to the developing embryo and then fetus via the umbilical cord. This cord houses a two-way "street" of blood vessels that connect the embryo/

fetus to a shared temporary organ called the placenta. The placenta, a pancake of tissue embedded in the mother's uterus, allows the exchange of oxygen, nutrients, and wastes between the mother's blood and the embryonic/fetal blood. If the mother has been drinking alcohol, it will move across the placenta and into the embryonic/fetal blood along with nutrients and oxygen.

As can drugs and viruses, alcohol can cause birth defects. It affects the development of many body systems, including the central nervous system, in a number of ways. Because it narrows blood vessels, alcohol affects the transfer of oxygen and nutrients to the embryo and fetus. It also affects the removal of wastes. It can cause cells to die, which results in abnormal development. Alcohol can also affect the way nerve cells develop and function. In addition, as the alcohol is internally processed, harmful by-products become concentrated in the developing brain.

> **Fetal alcohol disorders are 100 percent preventable if women do not drink while pregnant.**

The most vulnerable time is the first eight weeks of pregnancy, when the foundations of the major organ systems of the body are just beginning to develop. Some women do not even realize they are pregnant until well into this sensitive period. That is why it is important for women who are trying to get pregnant to stop drinking alcoholic beverages. In addition, women of childbearing age who drink alcohol and who are not trying to get pregnant should use contraception. As noted by the Substance Abuse and Mental Health Services Administration: "Any woman of childbearing age is at risk of having a child with an FASD if she drinks alcohol during pregnancy."[2] Fetal alcohol disorders are 100 percent preventable if women do not drink while pregnant.

Alcohol Labels and Warning Signs

A law requiring warning labels on alcoholic beverages was enacted in 1989. The purpose of the warning labels is to educate the public not only about the dangers of consuming alcohol during pregnancy but also about its general health risks. The label on every bottle of alcohol has two messages: "(1.) According to the Surgeon General, women should not drink alcoholic beverages during pregnancy because of the risk of birth defects. (2.) Consumption of alcoholic beverages impairs your ability to drive a car or operate machinery, and may cause health problems." In 1990 the words "Government Warning" were added to the label. Although the effectiveness of the label is unclear, as of 2010 it appeared on all alcohol, wine, and distilled spirits. Many states and localities also require that warning signs be posted wherever alcoholic beverages are sold.

What Are the Effects of Fetal Alcohol Disorders?

Some of the effects of alcohol on the embryo and fetus may appear immediately at birth, and some effects may appear only as the child grows and develops. These FASD effects last a lifetime and may be physical, cognitive, behavioral, and developmental.

The physical effects of fetal alcohol disorders include abnormal facial features. These deviations from normal facial structure include small eye openings, a flat midface, a short nose, a thin upper lip, and a smoothing out of the groove that runs from the nose to the upper lip. Appearing together, these facial characteristics are a sign of fetal alcohol syndrome. Sometimes these facial characteristics are subtle and hard to detect except by a physician trained in identifying them. Persons with subtle facial abnormalities may be diagnosed with partial fetal alcohol syndrome. Other types of physical effects of prenatal alcohol exposure include heart, skeletal, kidney, liver, and dental defects.

Brain Damage

Brain damage is the most serious physical effect of being exposed to alcohol before birth. Some babies born with fetal alcohol syndrome have a smaller-than-average head size. This condition, called microcephaly, may be present at birth or may develop during the first few years of life. Those with a fetal alcohol disorder also may have difficulties with speech, vision, and hearing. Other types of brain damage may result in cognitive and/or behavioral problems.

Cognitive refers to conscious intellectual activity, such as thinking, reasoning, or remembering. One measure of intellectual capacity is the intelligence quotient, or IQ. Average IQ is generally considered to fall within a range of 90 to 109; the average IQ of children with fetal alcohol

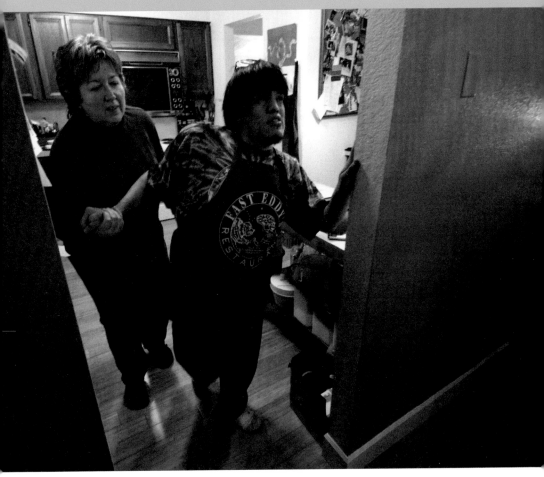

Fetal alcohol disorders begin in the womb but last a lifetime. Born with fetal alcohol syndrome, this young man struggles with developmental, cognitive, and physical impairments. His adoptive mother helps him walk through their house in Anchorage, Alaska.

syndrome is 68, which is considered mild mental retardation. Even in individuals with FASDs who do not have mental retardation, cognitive functions are generally affected negatively. The National Organization on Fetal Alcohol Syndrome notes that individuals with FASDs are challenged in their ability to perform daily life skills on their own, such as brushing their teeth or taking public transportation. In addition, persons with FASDs have problems with attention span and with understanding, processing, and remembering information.

The brain damage caused by alcohol exposure during prenatal de-

> **Some of the effects of alcohol on the embryo and fetus may appear immediately at birth, and some effects may appear only as the child grows and develops.**

velopment also results in behavioral problems. Persons with a fetal alcohol disorder are prone to hyperactivity, poor judgment, and impulsivity. They may lack fear and have no sense of boundaries. Many are troubled with low self-esteem.

Both physical and intellectual development is another problem area for persons with fetal alcohol disorders. Babies born with such disorders may be underweight and tiny, and they may exhibit extreme irritability. As they age, many FASD children eat and grow poorly. Some may have seizures and problems sleeping. Physical coordination is often difficult, including fine motor skills, such as working with the fingers, and gross motor skills, such as running and jumping.

Behavior Problems

Primary disabilities are challenges that stem directly from problems in the body's structure and function. Primary disabilities common with FASDs, such as mental retardation, hyperactivity, disruptiveness, and a disregard for rules, are due to brain damage that occurred during prenatal development. As the person with an FASD interacts with others and the environment, however, secondary disabilities may develop—disabilities that stem from their primary disabilities. These secondary disabilities include trouble with the law, inappropriate sexual behavior, alcohol and drug problems, mental health problems, problems with employment, and the inability to live independently.

Bonnie Buxton, an adoptive mother of a child with a fetal alcohol disorder, shares her thoughts on these disorders and on secondary disabilities in her insightful book *Damaged Angels*:

> The impulsiveness and poor judgment of children with FASD can only be controlled through diagnosis and loving support. . . . Those who grow up in a series of incompetent, uncaring, or abusive homes are likely to develop

secondary disabilities: dropping out of school, addiction, unemployment, homelessness, and trouble with the law. At risk of finding themselves in situations of violence and brutality, they may become victims themselves.[3]

According to the Substance Abuse and Mental Health Services Administration, 60 percent of people with an FASD who are age 12 and older have had trouble with the law. One reason is that those with such disorders have alcohol-damaged brains that distort how they think, feel, and behave. These distorted patterns of thinking may lead to criminal activity. Moreover, people with an FASD have other primary disabilities that may compound their risk of having trouble with the law. These problems may include difficulty handling social situations, poor judgment, impulsivity, and a disregard for authority.

> " **Brain damage is the most serious physical effect of being exposed to alcohol before birth.** "

Inappropriate sexual behavior is another example of a secondary disability of FASD. Buxton notes: "Girls with FASD often mature physically earlier than the norm, and many young alcohol-affected females delight in their precocious curves: they can't do math, but they *can* attract older men."[4]

Compounding the problem of early sexual maturation, people with a fetal alcohol disorder often have stunted emotional and social development, difficulties with impulsive behavior, and poor judgment. They are therefore at risk of exhibiting various inappropriate sexual behaviors, such as making unwanted sexual advances, exposing themselves in public, and making obscene phone calls. Girls with a fetal alcohol disorder are at high risk of having an unwanted pregnancy.

How Can a Person with a Fetal Alcohol Disorder Be Helped?

The damage wrought by alcohol on the fetus brings lifelong effects for which there is no cure. However, there are a variety of interventions that can help to increase well-being. In the classroom certain **teaching strat-**

egies may help students with fetal alcohol disorders. Making obvious the consequences of certain behaviors helps students with such disorders learn cause and effect. Having consistent and predictable routines helps them feel more secure and master day-to-day tasks. Breaking down instructions into small steps helps students with language or memory difficulties learn how to perform multistep tasks. Individualized education plans help target problem areas for students with these disorders and recommend various strategies or programs to help them reach personalized educational goals.

Medical professionals help those in the criminal justice system, such as lawyers, judges, corrections workers, and parole officers, understand FASD and how it affects individuals. In turn, this understanding helps those with a fetal alcohol disorder. For example, persons with such a disorder may not understand the legal process and may be suggestible during questioning. They may become confused or easily led to say things that are untrue. They may confess to crimes they did not commit. If convicted, they may not understand how to follow probation rules or follow orders in a jail or prison. Researchers Diane K. Fast and Julianne Conry note that "early recognition of the disabilities of people with FASDs may reduce the over-representation of this group in the CJS [criminal justice system], and better understanding of FASD should lead to improved support and fair treatment of individuals with FASDs."[5]

Some progress is being made in the understanding of fetal alcohol disorders in the legal system. Tyler Mills, an adult prison inmate with an FASD, was found not guilty of a crime in Wisconsin in 2009 due to mental defect caused by exposure to alcohol in the womb. This ruling provides Mills with psychological and medical treatment in a mental hospital instead of incarceration, a ruling that many find more appropriate than punishment. Clinical psychologist Natalie Novick Brown, who specializes in fetal alcohol disorders and the legal system, notes that this case and others show a growing positive awareness of the effect of these disorders on criminal behavior.

> **The damage wrought by alcohol on the fetus brings lifelong effects for which there is no cure.**

Supportive Home Environment

Quality care and stability of the home appear crucial to help those with a fetal alcohol disorder. Nevertheless, children born with an FASD have a biological mother who did not understand the dangers of drinking while pregnant or was addicted to alcohol and found herself unable to control her drinking. In addition to exposing her fetus to alcohol, the addicted mother may have exposed her fetus to other drugs as well. Thus, a positive and stable family environment may not be a reality for many children with a fetal alcohol disorder.

Even in supportive and nurturing home environments, FASD children provide daily and possibly overwhelming challenges for their parents and other family members. Research results on fetal alcohol disorders are only beginning to provide insight into specific ways in which parents and other family members can help those with such a disorder. However, families can seek help to learn various techniques, such as skill-building practice, behavior management techniques, and other methods of positive parent-child interactions, in their quest to support their FASD child and find the support they need as well.

What Are Fetal Alcohol Disorders?

66It [FAS] has affected my life in several ways. I explain it this way to my friends, my body is 37 years old, but my brain is 20 years old.99

—Rob A., who in 1973 was the first infant diagnosed with fetal alcohol syndrome in the United States.

66When Zach was a baby, I started wondering if something was wrong with him. He didn't reach the same milestones as other children. He rolled instead of crawled, was uncoordinated when he tried to walk, and by age three his speech was so garbled I couldn't understand anything he said.99

—Lorrie H., a single parent of a child with a fetal alcohol disorder.

Fetal alcohol disorders are incurable birth defects caused by alcohol exposure during prenatal development. Fetal alcohol disorders range in their severity and effects, so the phrase "fetal alcohol spectrum disorders" (FASD) has been coined to refer to the entire group. The various effects seen under the FASD "umbrella" include growth deficiencies, brain dysfunctions, distinctive facial features, and structural birth defects.

Fetal alcohol exposure results in a spectrum of disorders because many factors are involved in their development: the amount and timing of alcohol consumption by a pregnant woman, the susceptibility of the fetus to the effects of alcohol, and the genetic characteristics and age of the woman while pregnant. For example, research results published in the October 2010 issue of the journal *Alcoholism: Clinical and Experimental Research* show that a mother's age when pregnant is important in the development of these disorders. Children born to drinking mothers 30 years of age and older were more susceptible to the effects of alcohol during prenatal development than children born to younger drinking mothers. Nonetheless, the children of younger drinking mothers are not immune to the effects of alcohol during their pre-birth development. Although no exact relationship has been determined between the amount and timing of drinking and the effects on the fetus, no safe level of alcohol consumption during pregnancy has been found for pregnant women of any age.

Separating Fetal Alcohol Disorders from Other Problems

When a child exhibits physiological and behavioral characteristics that cause concern for parents, teachers, and possibly the law, how do those involved determine what is wrong? Does the child have a short attention span, difficulty remembering, or trouble completing everyday tasks, such as getting dressed? Is he or she belligerent, forgetful, or hostile? Is growth delayed or cognitive function impaired? Not all these problems in every child are caused by a fetal alcohol disorder. Additionally, not all problems in FASD children are due to the disorder alone. Persons with these disorders often have other conditions or disorders too, such as bipolar disorder, autism, or schizophrenia.

> " **Fetal alcohol disorders are incurable birth defects caused by alcohol exposure during prenatal development.** "

Differentiating between fetal alcohol disorders and other disorders can be extremely challenging, as can be distinguishing among FASDs. Accounts from adoptive parents of children later diagnosed with a fetal alcohol disorder often include the words "I knew from the start that there was something different about my child." Many turn to the Internet to find answers. Often these parents "see" their child in what they read about fetal alcohol disorders. But often they see their child in descriptions of other disorders, too. However, information helps give direction and is a beginning to the diagnostic process.

Another beginning step is to find out whether the biological mother of the child drank alcohol during pregnancy. Sometimes this cannot be determined for certain. Either way, determining whether a child has an FASD and distinguishing among possible FASDs usually requires a team of health and education professionals.

Screening Tests for Prenatal Alcohol Exposure

A medical screening test is a procedure done to identify the presence of a specific disease in a person that has no symptoms of that disease. As yet, there are no widely used screening tests for FASDs, but researchers noted in the July 2010 issue of the journal *Developmental Neuroscience* that a screening test for infants to detect exposure to alcohol in the womb has been developed.

The authors of the article, researchers from Georgetown University Medical Center in Washington, DC, explain that if a fetus was exposed to alcohol in late pregnancy, some of the breakdown products of the alcohol are present in the first bowel movement of the infant. The test can detect these chemical compounds if present. However, this test is able to identify only infants exposed to alcohol in a late stage of pregnancy.

Alcohol breakdown products in the first stool of an infant are an example of a biological marker. Biological markers are measurable products produced by an organism that can be used in assessments of health and physiology. Researchers are working to find other biological markers that could be used in the early detection of prenatal alcohol exposure.

Diagnosing Fetal Alcohol Disorders

According to the Substance Abuse and Mental Health Services Administration, getting an early, accurate diagnosis is critical to providing FASD children with effective treatment to help reduce the severity of disabilities. Although some of the effects of an FASD may seem the same as effects of other conditions, treatment or intervention may not be the same because the underlying cause is different. Thus, accurate diagnosis is key.

Francis Perry, an adult living with a fetal alcohol disorder, relates how important diagnosis was to him: "Getting diagnosed was like a weight lifted off my shoulders. Now I know I have a problem and that I am not the problem. Before I was diagnosed . . . all I had were feelings of hatred anger, bitterness, resentment and fear . . . constantly questioning my existence and swamped with thoughts of suicide. I now . . . know what my limitations are."[6]

Fetal alcohol spectrum disorders include fetal alcohol syndrome (FAS), partial fetal alcohol syndrome, alcohol-related neurodevelopmental disorder, and alcohol-related birth defects. Fetal alcohol syndrome is the most severe effect of alcohol on the fetus, with the exception of fetal death, and is the easiest to diagnose. The other fetal alcohol disorders may prove more of a diagnostic challenge.

Fetal Alcohol Syndrome

Children with fetal alcohol syndrome have patterns of problems in three areas: abnormal facial characteristics, slowed growth, and central nervous system abnormalities. The three abnormal facial characteristics of this syndrome that are most important in diagnosing the condition are a missing groove above the upper lip, small eye openings, and a thin upper lip. However, an individual with FAS may also have other abnormal facial characteristics, including a flattened nasal bridge, which is the portion of the nose between the eyes; ear malformations; a short, up-turned nose; and a small web of tissue overlapping the inner corners of the eyes.

> Differentiating between fetal alcohol disorders and other disorders can be extremely challenging, as can be distinguishing among FASDs.

Slowed growth and central nervous system abnormalities are also hallmarks of fetal alcohol syndrome. Children with this syndrome may be shorter than others their age and may have been small at birth. They may also weigh less than their peers. The central nervous system abnormalities may include a small head and brain, mental retardation, seizures, hyperactivity, developmental delays such as speech and language problems, attention deficits, learning and memory impairments, poor coordination, poor muscle control, and poor sucking characteristics as an infant.

Other Disorders on the Spectrum

Most children exposed to alcohol during their prenatal development do not exhibit all the characteristics of full-blown fetal alcohol syndrome. Instead they show a range of less-specific physical changes and neurodevelopmental problems.

Children who were exposed to alcohol in the womb and have all the characteristics of fetal alcohol syndrome but who have normal growth patterns have partial FAS. The partial FAS child has the same cognitive and behavioral challenges as a person with full FAS.

Children who were exposed to alcohol in the womb and do not have facial characteristics typical of FAS, but who have severe central nervous system dysfunction, have alcohol-related neurodevelopmental disorder. In addition, some children with this disorder may have more serious problems with critical cognitive skills called "executive function" than those with full FAS. These skills include writing, starting and finishing work, solving problems, and controlling emotions. Another of these skills is remembering. Morgan Fawcett, a 17-year-old from the Tlingit Indian Tribe of Alaska, has turned his poor memory into an asset. The teenager plays the flute, and each song he plays is an original composition because he cannot remember the music to any songs.

> "According to the Substance Abuse and Mental Health Services Administration, getting an early, accurate diagnosis is critical to providing FASD children with effective treatment to help reduce the severity of disabilities."

Children who were exposed to alcohol in the womb and do not have all the neurodevelopmental problems of the other FASDs, but who have one or more birth defects, have alcohol-related birth defects. The Institute of Medicine lists a wide range of birth defects that can be caused by prenatal alcohol exposure. Some of the birth defects most commonly associated with fetal alcohol exposure are malformations of the heart, bones, or kidneys, and may involve abnormal development of structures associated with vision and hearing.

Effects of Alcohol on Prenatal Development

The first trimester of pregnancy is a period of rapid development of the embryo and fetus. It is a time in which the developing organism is most vulnerable to structural defects because the body's foundation is being laid down. The effects of alcohol during this time were the topic of an October 2010 *Pediatrics* article. Researchers from England and Australia published the first known study using population data to examine the relationship between the amount, pattern, and timing of prenatal alcohol exposure and birth defects. The researchers' analysis of the data revealed an association between heavy maternal drinking during the first three months of pregnancy and a fourfold increased risk of birth defects. They found that the most frequently occurring birth defects caused by heavy maternal drinking during the first trimester were structural defects of the heart.

> " The second and third trimesters are a time of fetal maturation and growth. The fetal brain is the most sensitive of all the organs to alcohol during this time. "

The second and third trimesters are a time of fetal maturation and growth. The fetal brain is the most sensitive of all the organs to alcohol during this time. Because it has a high density of blood vessels, it receives more of the alcohol than other organs. The National Institutes of Health notes, however, that some regions of the brain are more sensitive to the effects of alcohol than others during prenatal development. Regions that are particularly vulnerable include the frontal cortex, which is associated with judgment, impulse control, and functions such as remembering and solving problems; the hippocampus, which is associated with emotion and memory; the corpus callosum, which connects the right and left sides of the brain and allows nerve impulses to pass back and forth; and various parts of the cerebellum, which controls coordination and movement.

How Developmental Processes Are Altered

Scientists are still learning about how alcohol causes birth defects in the embryo and fetus and interferes with proper development. It has been determined however, that many genes that direct development are altered by alcohol exposure. Alterations in the genes result in alterations in the developmental processes, including cell migration, growth, and differentiation. Cell migration is a process in which certain cells move to specific locations in a developing organism. These movements are critical to proper development, and errors in cell migration result in serious developmental effects. Cell differentiation is a process in which less-specialized cells become more-specialized cells. For example, during development some cells will differentiate into heart cells while others will become brain cells. Once again, errors in this crucial developmental process result in serious developmental effects.

The Scope of the Problem

According to the National Institutes of Health, alcohol is the leading known environmental cause of birth defects. Forty thousand infants—about 1 percent of all infants born each year in the United States—enter the world with a fetal alcohol disorder because they were exposed to alcohol in the womb.

The Native American population has a particularly high rate of FASD births, reaching as high as 2.5 percent in some tribes. The Substance Abuse and Mental Health Services Administration attributes the high FASD rate among Native American newborns not only to the high rate of alcoholism in the adult female Native American population, but also to the high rate of poverty and poor access to health care. In addition, points out William J. Szlemko and colleagues from the Tri-Ethnic Center for Prevention Research at Colorado State University, alcohol prevention programs for Native Americans are difficult to develop. Says Szlemko, "With over 500 federally recognized tribes, with each its own history, culture, and traditions . . . preventions that work for one tribe may be inappropriate or even counterproductive in another."[7]

Fetal alcohol disorders affect infants all over the world. The National Institutes of Health states that the rate of these disorders is more common in some other parts of the world than in the United States, especially in areas in which heavy drinking is the norm, such as the Western Cape province of South Africa and Moscow, Russia. The Substance Abuse and Mental Health Services Administration's FASD Center for Excellence recognizes fetal alcohol disorders as a global issue and works toward decreasing the incidence of fetal alcohol disorders worldwide.

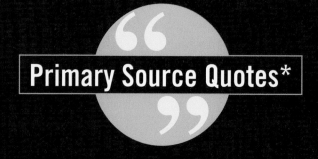
What Are Fetal Alcohol Disorders?

"Though FAS is a well-recognized disorder, it is still in its infancy in medical literature."

—Mahendra Kumar Banakar, Nirvana Swamy Kudlur, and Sanju George, "Fetal Alcohol Spectrum Disorder (FASD)," *Indian Journal of Pediatrics*, November 2009.

The authors are clinical researchers practicing in the United Kingdom.

"Lack of recognition of FASD is remarkable given that economic analysis finds that the full FAS, one condition on the larger fetal alcohol spectrum, is the most costly birth defect in the U.S."

—Heather Carmichael Olson, Rosalind Oti, Julie Gelo, and Sharon Beck, "'Family Matters': Fetal Alcohol Spectrum Disorders and the Family," *Developmental Disabilities Research Reviews*, August 1, 2009.

The authors are clinical researchers practicing in Seattle, Washington.

* Editor's Note: While the definition of a primary source can be narrowly or broadly defined, for the purposes of Compact Research, a primary source consists of: 1) results of original research presented by an organization or researcher; 2) eyewitness accounts of events, personal experience, or work experience; 3) first-person editorials offering pundits' opinions; 4) government officials presenting political plans and/or policies; 5) representatives of organizations presenting testimony or policy.

66 Failure to diagnose an individual as having a brain damaged by alcohol, malnutrition, head trauma or any other misfortune is widespread in the medical community. **99**

—Charles Huffine, "Psychiatry and FASD," *Iceberg Newsletter*, March 2010. http://fasiceberg.org.

Huffine is a practicing child and adolescent psychiatrist in Seattle, Washington, and a specialist in fetal alcohol disorders.

66 Correctly diagnosing a child with FAS before age 6 can have a protective influence, decreasing the odds that he or she will suffer severe secondary disabilities in adolescence and adulthood. **99**

—Mary C. Boyce, "A Better Future for Baby: Stemming the Tide of Fetal Alcohol Syndrome," *Journal of Family Practice*, June 2010.

Boyce is a physician in the Department of Family and Community Medicine and Wesley Family Medicine Residency, University of Kansas School of Medicine, Wichita.

66 Signs of FASD don't always appear at birth. **99**

—HealthLink BC, "Alcohol Effects on a Fetus," May 5, 2009. www.healthlinkbc.ca.

HealthLink BC is a service of the British Columbia Ministry of Health in Canada.

66 FASDs are considered both medical conditions and developmental disabilities. **99**

—National Task Force on Fetal Alcohol Syndrome and Fetal Alcohol Effect, "A Call to Action: Advancing Essential Services and Research on Fetal Alcohol Spectrum Disorders," March 2009. www.cdc.gov.

The National Task Force on Fetal Alcohol Syndrome and Fetal Alcohol Effect includes scientists, clinicians, and persons providing services to those with FASDs.

❝Fetal alcohol syndrome (FAS) is the most common cause of preventable mental retardation in the United States.❞

—Valborg L. Kvigne et al., "Characteristics of Children Whose Siblings Have Fetal Alcohol Syndrome or Incomplete Fetal Alcohol Syndrome," *Pediatrics*, March 2009.

The authors are researchers and experts in the field of fetal alcohol disorders.

❝My differences are hidden and that's a real pain, because it is easy to judge a person by what you see.❞

—Liz Kulp, *Braided Cord: Tough Times In and Out*. Minneapolis: Better Endings New Beginnings, 2010.

Kulp is an adult with a fetal alcohol disorder who was diagnosed in her teens.

What Are Fetal Alcohol Disorders?

- Fetal alcohol disorders range from mild **intellectual and behavioral problems** to extreme disorders that lead to profound disabilities or **premature death**.

- Fetal alcohol disorders are not hereditary; they are **100 percent preventable**. The sole cause is prenatal alcohol exposure.

- According to the Centers for Disease Control and Prevention, for every diagnosed case of fetal alcohol syndrome, there are believed to be **four times** as many cases of fetal alcohol disorders, many of which are undiagnosed.

- Researchers from the University of New Mexico and Wayne State University studied the prevalence of fetal alcohol disorders in the Lazio region of Italy, where drinking daily with meals is commonplace. Results indicate that the prevalence of fetal alcohol disorders there was **2 to 4 percent**; it is approximately **1 percent** in the United States.

- Research on the characteristics of Northern Plains American Indian maternal grandmothers revealed that **93 percent** of those who had grandchildren with fetal alcohol syndrome and **78 percent** of those who had grandchildren with partial fetal alcohol syndrome were documented alcohol users.

- Of the children heavily exposed to alcohol before birth, about **40 percent** are estimated to exhibit fetal alcohol disorders, with **4 percent** affected by full-blown fetal alcohol syndrome.

Signs of Fetal Alcohol Syndrome

Fetal alcohol syndrome is the most severe of the fetal alcohol disorders. Children with fetal alcohol syndrome have distinctive facial features, growth deficiency, and central nervous system abnormalities. These and other characteristics, along with the mother's drinking history, help doctors identify children born with fetal alcohol syndrome.

Fetal alcohol syndrome may include:

- Distinctive facial features, including small eyes; an exceptionally thin upper lip; a short, upturned nose; and a smooth skin surface between the nose and upper lip
- Heart defects
- Deformities of joints, limbs, and fingers
- Slow physical growth before and after birth
- Vision difficulties or hearing problems
- Small head circumference and brain size (microcephaly)
- Poor coordination
- Sleep problems
- Mental retardation and delayed development
- Learning disorders
- Abnormal behaviors, such as a short attention span, hyperactivity, poor impulse control, extreme nervousness and anxiety

Source: The Mayo Clinic, "Fetal Alcohol Syndrome: Symptoms," May 22, 2009. www.mayoclinic.com.

- Russia has very high rates of alcoholism; the prevalence of children with fetal alcohol syndrome in Russian orphanages is estimated to be 15 per 1,000, or **1.5 percent**.

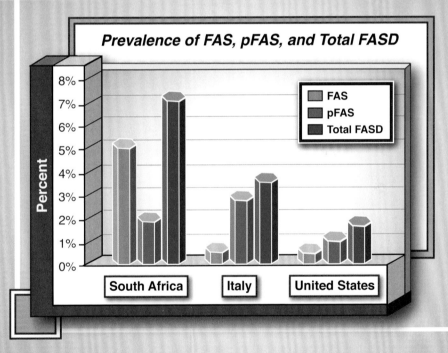

Prevalence of Fetal Alcohol Disorders

Estimating the prevalence of fetal alcohol disorders—not only in the United States but also in other countries—is challenging. Many researchers believe that the prevalence is underestimated. A 2009 study estimated the prevalence of these disorders among schoolchildren in South Africa, Italy, and the United States. The study looked at fetal alcohol syndrome (FAS), and a variation known as partial fetal alcohol syndrome (pFAS), and also gave results for the full spectrum of disorders, known as fetal alcohol spectrum disorders (FASDs). Researchers noted that high levels of alcohol consumption among women in parts of South Africa helped explain higher rates of fetal alcohol disorders in that country.

Prevalence of FAS, pFAS, and Total FASD

Source: Philip A. May et al., "Prevalence and Epidemiologic Characteristics of FASD from Various Research Methods with an Emphasis on Recent In-School Studies," *Developmental Disabilities Research Reviews*, vol. 15, 2009.

- Research data suggest that women who give birth to a child with fetal alcohol syndrome are **800 times** more likely to give birth to subsequent children with the syndrome than are women who have never given birth to a child with the syndrome.

Comparing Fetal Alcohol Disorders with Other Birth Defects

According to the National Organization on Fetal Alcohol Syndrome, fetal alcohol disorders affect about 40,000 newborns each year. The spectrum of these disorders, abbreviated as FASDs, affect far more infants annually than Down syndrome (birth defects resulting from a genetic problem), spina bifida (birth defects of the spine), and muscular dystrophy (birth defects involving the muscles).

Estimated Annual Number of Cases of FASDs and Other Birth Defects in the United States

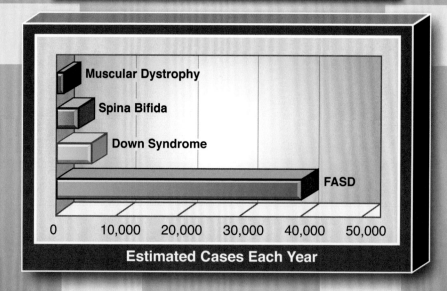

Source: National Organization on Fetal Alcohol Syndrome, "FASD: What Everyone Should Know," www.nofas.org.

- Each year there are **four times** as many infants born with fetal alcohol disorders as there are infants born with muscular dystrophy, spina bifida, and Down syndrome together.

- **Fifteen out of every 100** women of childbearing age do not know that drinking alcoholic beverages during pregnancy is dangerous.

What Is the Cause of Fetal Alcohol Disorders?

❝It's not easy to admit that I hurt my son. . . . Back in 1979, I was 18, had moved out of my parents' home . . . and had quit school to work. At 23, after a brief affair, I got pregnant. I was excited about the baby but continued drinking and partying with my friends. I didn't think about the consequences.❞

—Lorrie Hundel, mother of Zach, who has a fetal alcohol disorder.

❝If a woman is drinking alcohol during pregnancy, it is never too late to stop. The sooner a woman stops drinking, the better it will be for both her baby and herself.❞

—Centers for Disease Control and Prevention.

❝With every sip that Debbie Crowell took from the icy can of Budweiser," writes *Tucson Citizen* reporter Gabrielle Fimbres, "the tiny baby growing inside her belly became more and more drunk. Crowell, 29, knew that as a pregnant woman, she shouldn't drink. But she had drunk during some of her six pregnancies before this one, and each of those babies looked OK to her. So she drank. . . . As Crowell got more and more drunk, so did her child, Sabrina."[8] Sabrina started having seizures when she was about six months old; doctors suspected fetal alcohol syndrome. Another of Crowell's children, found to have brain damage, was diagnosed with the same disorder at age three.

Drinking During Pregnancy

As Crowell now knows, fetal alcohol disorders are caused by maternal drinking during pregnancy. Alcohol can have devastating effects on a developing embryo and fetus, the worst of which is death and subsequent miscarriage. And if a developing embryo or fetus does not die from alcohol exposure, it may develop a fetal alcohol disorder. Fetal alcohol disorders, more technically called fetal alcohol spectrum disorders, are a range of incurable disabilities in the areas of intelligence, cognition, growth, and development.

Alcohol and Prenatal Development

During prenatal development, alcohol not only interferes with critical cell processes such as taking in nutrients and eliminating wastes, but it can also affect genes—the hereditary material—and the developmental processes that genes direct. These dangerous effects can begin immediately in a pregnancy. If alcohol is circulating in the mother's blood, it reaches the pre-embryo as early as the first week of development, when the dividing ball of cells is making its way through the mother's uterine tube on its way to the uterus. Alcohol can affect any of these cells, which all play critical roles in the future development of the embryo and fetus. In addition, alcohol could delay implantation of the pre-embryo in the uterine wall, which would delay the genetically orchestrated developmental processes that follow.

> **Alcohol can have devastating effects on a developing embryo and fetus, the worst of which is death and subsequent miscarriage.**

Weeks two through eight of development are the embryonic stage, a crucial and sensitive time in development. During this period, cells divide, move, and differentiate. Some cells become heart cells, while others become brain cells, for example. By the end of the eighth week, most of the body systems are functional even though the embryo is only about 1 inch (2.54cm) long. And as tissues and organs develop during this period, they are highly sensitive to the toxic effects of alcohol. Structural changes can occur to the face, which forms during the embryonic period, as well as to the heart, brain, and a host of other tissues and organs.

The fetal period begins at the ninth week of development and continues until birth. The fetal period is one primarily of maturation and growth of the organs that have already developed. The sensory organs, such as the eyes and ears, finish their development. However, the central nervous system, which includes the brain and spinal cord, continues development during the fetal period and does not finish its development and maturation until well after birth. Thus, alcohol can damage the brain and other central nervous system structures and connections throughout pregnancy.

> **Alcohol can damage the brain and other central nervous system structures and connections throughout pregnancy.**

How Much Is Too Much During Pregnancy?

The Centers for Disease Control and Prevention (CDC) states that no amount of alcohol is safe to consume at any time during pregnancy. In addition, drinking any kind of alcohol, whether it is in the form of beer, wine, or spirits, is unsafe during pregnancy.

Researchers from the United Kingdom, in a study published in October 2010 in the *Journal of Epidemiology and Community Health*, conclude that light drinking during pregnancy—1 to 2 drinks per week or per occasion—did not result in cognitive or behavioral deficits in children up to 5 years of age. The researchers have no data on children older than 5, however, and the effects of fetal alcohol exposure often show up in school-aged children when none was evident earlier. Previously, the UK researchers had published similar data on the same children up to 3 years of age.

After reviewing the data, the CDC has *not* changed its recommendation and advises all pregnant women to abstain from alcohol completely. The Fetal Alcohol Spectrum Disorders Study Group made this statement on light drinking during pregnancy:

The consensus recommendation of the hundreds of scientists and clinical investigators, who study Fetal Alcohol Spectrum Disorders, along with public health officials around the world, is very clear—a woman should abstain from drinking during pregnancy as part of an overall program of good prenatal care that includes good nutrition, adequate exercise, sufficient rest, and proper prenatal health care.[9]

Pregnant women are not the only group who should abstain from alcohol to avoid exposing an embryo or fetus to alcohol's dangerous effects. Women who are planning on becoming pregnant and sexually active women who are of childbearing age and not using contraception should abstain from drinking alcohol. The first weeks and months of a pregnancy are an extremely sensitive developmental time for the embryo and fetus, and women who do not know they are pregnant and who drink could unwittingly harm their future child's health in devastating ways.

Drinking During the Childbearing Years

The CDC has surveyed thousands of women of childbearing age since 1991 on their alcohol use and binge drinking—consuming 5 or more drinks on any one occasion. Research results reported in the CDC's 2009 report "Alcohol Use Among Pregnant and Nonpregnant Women of Childbearing Age" revealed that the prevalence of alcohol use and binge drinking among pregnant and nonpregnant women did not change substantially over the years since the surveys were begun in 1991.

Overall, the CDC results showed that about 12 percent of pregnant women admitted they consumed alcohol when they were pregnant. Nearly 2 percent said they engaged in binge drinking while pregnant. These percentages could be higher in reality, since the results are self-reported and some pregnant women may have chosen not to reveal their drinking behaviors.

Nonpregnant women of childbearing age reported a much higher prevalence of drinking than pregnant women. Over half (54 percent) of nonpregnant women of childbearing age who were surveyed by the CDC reported alcohol use in the month prior to the survey, and slightly over 12 percent reported binge drinking. These high percentages of alcohol use and binge drinking in women of childbearing age is a public health concern, because these women may become pregnant, not know that they are pregnant, and continue with their usual drinking patterns. The CDC notes that only 40 percent of women realize that they are pregnant 4 weeks into their pregnancy, while 4 critical weeks of embryonic development have already taken place. Additionally, 60 percent of women continue their pregnancy past 4 weeks unaware and may unknowingly expose their embryo and fetus to alcohol in the womb.

Screening for Alcohol Misuse

Many tests exist to determine whether a person needs help with his or her drinking. These tests screen for at-risk, heavy, or harmful drinking, and they include in-depth interviews, biochemical tests, and questionnaires. The first alcohol screening test for pregnant women was the T-ACE questionnaire, which was developed in 1989 and is still in use today. It consists of four questions that focus on the level of alcohol tolerance, the annoyance of others to the drinking, the perception of needing to cut down on one's drinking, and the use of a drink as an eye-opener in the morning. Other alcohol screening tests for pregnant women exist, too. All are designed to be administered by physicians caring for women of childbearing age in an effort to reduce the development of fetal alcohol disorders.

> " The data on teen contraceptive use and unplanned pregnancy, coupled with the data on female teen alcohol use, reveal an at-risk population for fetal alcohol exposure and FASDs. "

Unplanned Pregnancies and Fetal Alcohol Disorders

Unplanned or unintended pregnancies are those that occur sooner than desired or those that are unwanted. Unplanned pregnancies occur either because contraception was not used during sexual intercourse, it was not used properly, or it failed.

Women who did not intend to become pregnant are less likely to know they are pregnant early in the pregnancy than women who are trying to become pregnant and are monitoring the process. The CDC notes that prenatal care is often delayed in unplanned pregnancies, which puts the mother and fetus at risk not only for poor health outcomes but also for unknowingly consuming alcohol during the pregnancy, especially the first trimester. In addition, teens are at higher risk for unplanned pregnancy than are other age groups of women.

Teen Pregnancies and Fetal Alcohol Disorders

Every two years the CDC conducts a nationwide survey called the Youth Risk Behavior Surveillance. The 2009 survey results, published by the CDC in 2010, show that nearly half (about 46 percent) of high school girls reported having had sexual intercourse. Nearly 36 percent reported that they were currently sexually active. Only about half of these young women's partners (54 percent) used a condom during sex, while less than one-quarter (23 percent) of the women used birth control pills.

These data help explain why nearly two-thirds of pregnancies in teens under the age of 18 are unplanned, which is higher than the national average. About half of all pregnancies to teens aged 18 and 19 are unplanned, a proportion equivalent to the national average. In 2008, 435,000 children were born to teens aged 15 to 19, according to the CDC and the National Center for Health Statistics.

> **All women of childbearing age should be told that no safe level of alcohol consumption in pregnancy has been established.**

The Youth Risk Behavior Surveillance also collects data on alcohol use. The 2009 survey results show that about three-fourths (74 percent) of high-school-age girls said they had consumed alcohol sometime previously, and nearly 43 percent of high-school-age girls reported consuming alcohol within 1 month of the survey. Nearly one-fourth (over 23 percent) engaged in binge drinking within the month prior to the survey.

These data on teen contraceptive use and unplanned pregnancy, coupled with the data on female teen alcohol use, reveal an at-risk population for fetal alcohol exposure and FASDs. In addition, Planned Parenthood notes that one-third of pregnant teenage girls do not receive adequate prenatal medical care. Without prenatal care, pregnant teens may be unaware that alcohol can harm their developing fetus and that their drinking can leave their child with lifelong disabilities.

Preventing Drinking in Women of Childbearing Age

Researchers at the Emory University Maternal Substance Abuse and Child Development Study cite many misconceptions about fetal alcohol spectrum disorders. One of these misconceptions is that mothers who drink during pregnancy are callous and indifferent to the damage they might be causing to their unborn child, and that they have an easy choice to stop drinking. The medical professionals at Emory note that alcoholic women need help with their addiction and with birth control. In addition, many pregnant alcoholic women use multiple drugs and also need help with their addiction to drugs such as cocaine and heroin.

Bruce Ritchie, the husband of a woman who drank during her pregnancy with their son, adds a personal dimension to the discussion on pregnant, alcoholic women:

> When people say unkind things about birth moms who have children with FASD, it is usually out of ignorance of the nature of addictions, frustration about the unnecessary injury to a child and/or a feeling of helplessness. . . . Nobody chooses to become addicted to alcohol or tobacco just as nobody chooses to get cancer. Whether the disease comes from genetics or environmental toxins (physical or psychological) is irrelevant. These are medical/biological issues that have to be dealt with, not moral decisions.[10]

For the general population of women of childbearing age, brief advice and counseling appear to be effective in reducing the risk of fetal alcohol disorders. The CDC suggests that all women of childbearing age be screened for alcohol use by their physicians. Those who use alcohol should be counseled *before* they become pregnant about the adverse effects of alcohol during pregnancy. In addition, all women of childbearing age should be told that no safe level of alcohol consumption in pregnancy has been established.

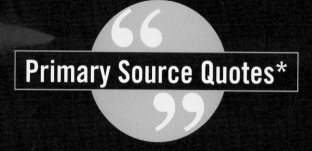

What Is the Cause of
Fetal Alcohol Disorders?

66 **Alcohol consumption during pregnancy is a risk factor for poor birth outcomes, including fetal alcohol syndrome, birth defects, and low birth weight.** 99

—Clark Denny et al., "Alcohol Use Among Pregnant and Nonpregnant Women of Childbearing Age—United States, 1991–2005," *Morbidity and Mortality Weekly Report*, May 22, 2009.

The authors are researchers with the National Center on Birth Defects and Developmental Disabilities of the Centers for Disease Control and Prevention.

66 **Every pregnancy is different. Drinking alcohol may hurt one baby more than another.** 99

—National Institute on Alcohol Abuse and Alcoholism, "Drinking and Your Pregnancy," 2009. http://pubs.niaaa.nih.gov.

The National Institute on Alcohol Abuse and Alcoholism is part of the National Institutes of Health.

* Editor's Note: While the definition of a primary source can be narrowly or broadly defined, for the purposes of Compact Research, a primary source consists of: 1) results of original research presented by an organization or researcher; 2) eyewitness accounts of events, personal experience, or work experience; 3) first-person editorials offering pundits' opinions; 4) government officials presenting political plans and/or policies; 5) representatives of organizations presenting testimony or policy.

Primary Source Quotes

❝ Reliance on self-report measures makes it difficult to obtain accurate information regarding the quantity, timing, frequency, and pattern of maternal alcohol intake. ❞

—Michelle Todorow, Timothy E, Moore, and Gideon Koren, "Investigating the Effects of Low to Moderate Levels of Prenatal Alcohol Exposure on Child Behaviour: A Critical Review," *Journal of Population Therapeutics and Clinical Pharmacology*, October 18, 2010.

Todorow, Moore, and Koren are clinical researchers from York University and the Hospital for Sick Children, both in Toronto, Canada.

❝ The earliest stages of life are periods of great vulnerability to the adverse effects of alcohol. ❞

—National Institutes of Health, "Fetal Alcohol Spectrum Disorders Fact Sheet," July 2007. www.nih.gov .

The National Institutes of Health is a governmental organization that seeks to determine basic knowledge about living systems and apply that knowledge to improve health.

❝ There is no proof that heavy drinking by the father can cause FASDs. ❞

—March of Dimes, "Quick Reference Fact Sheets: Drinking Alcohol During Pregnancy," 2010. www.marchofdimes.com.

The primary focus of the March of Dimes is improving the health of babies.

❝ Mothers are not the only ones who can prevent FAS. The father's role is also important in helping the woman abstain from drinking alcohol during pregnancy. ❞

—Wheeler Clinic's Connecticut Clearinghouse, "Fetal Alcohol Syndrome," 2010. www.ctclearinghouse.org.

The Wheeler Clinic provides behavioral health services for children, adolescents, adults, and families.

"A strong predictor of alcohol use during pregnancy is alcohol use levels prior to pregnancy."

—R. Louise Floyd et al., "Prevention of Fetal Alcohol Spectrum Disorders," *Developmental Disabilities Research Reviews*, August 1, 2009.

Floyd and her colleagues are researchers with the Centers for Disease Control and Prevention and at the Semel Institute for Neuroscience and Human Behavior at the University of California–Los Angeles.

"Women should avoid alcohol entirely while pregnant or trying to conceive because damage can occur in the earliest weeks of pregnancy, even before a woman knows that she is pregnant."

—American Congress of Obstetricians and Gynecologists, "Alcohol and Pregnancy: Know the Facts," February 6, 2008. www.acog.org.

The American Congress of Obstetricians and Gynecologists is a leading organization of professionals who provide health care for women.

"All drinks with alcohol can hurt an unborn baby."

—National Center on Birth Defects and Developmental Disabilities, "What Every Woman Should Know About Alcohol and Pregnancy," Centers for Disease Control and Prevention, April 27, 2009. www.cdc.gov.

The National Center on Birth Defects and Developmental Disabilities is a division of the Centers for Disease Control and Prevention, the nation's premier health protection office.

What Is the Cause of Fetal Alcohol Disorders?

- A survey of pediatricians reported in the journal *Pediatrics* revealed that only **13 percent** routinely discussed the risks of drinking during pregnancy with their adolescent patients.

- The National Organization on Fetal Alcohol Syndrome states that an estimated **40 percent** of the 60 million US women in their childbearing years (15 to 44) do not practice contraception.

- **Half** of all pregnancies in the United States are unplanned.

- According to the Center for Substance Abuse Prevention, **1 in 9 pregnant** women **binge drink** during the first trimester.

- Research results published in a 2009 article in the journal *Alcohol* revealed that children who were exposed to high doses of alcohol before birth were almost **2 times** as likely to have been exposed to narcotic opiates and **3.3 times** as likely to have been exposed to amphetamines compared with children who were not exposed to alcohol before birth.

- Results of a study published in 2010 on the assessment of the benefits of universal screening for alcohol use during pregnancy revealed that preventing future births of children with fetal alcohol syndrome in the binge drinking population would save an estimated **$48 billion** in direct costs and lifetime productivity losses.

Alcohol Use by Pregnant and Nonpregnant Women

The prevalence of alcohol use by pregnant and nonpregnant women in recent years has changed very little. Approximately 12 percent of women use alcohol and about 2 percent engage in binge drinking, behaviors that put the fetus at risk for fetal alcohol disorders. In addition, over half of nonpregnant women who are of childbearing age use alcohol, and about 12 percent binge drink. These women could unknowingly be pregnant and risk exposing their fetuses to these disorders.

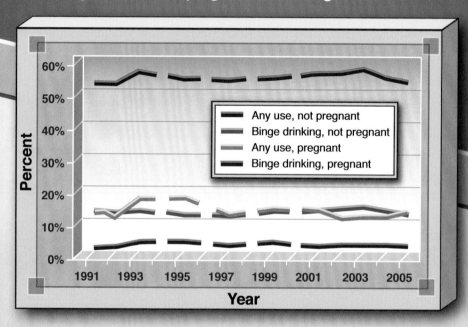

Self-reported alcohol use and binge drinking by pregnant and nonpregnant women aged 18–44

Legend:
- Any use, not pregnant
- Binge drinking, not pregnant
- Any use, pregnant
- Binge drinking, pregnant

Y-axis: Percent (0%–60%)
X-axis: Year (1991, 1993, 1995, 1997, 1999, 2001, 2003, 2005)

Note: Binge drinking is defined as five or more drinks on at least one occasion.

Source: Centers for Disease Control and Prevention, "Alcohol Use Among Pregnant and Nonpregnant Women of Childbearing Age—United States, 1991–2005," *Morbidity and Mortality Weekly Report*, May 22, 2009. www.cdc.gov.

- The Connecticut branch of the National Organization on Fetal Alcohol Syndrome reveals that about **15 percent** of women do not know that drinking alcohol during pregnancy is dangerous to the fetus.

Drinking Patterns Show Risk to Fetus

Some women of childbearing age drink more than others. One study published in 2009 found that college-educated women drank more than women with less education and that heavier use was higher among 18-to-24-year-old women than other age groups. Women of childbearing age who drink are at greater risk of exposing a fetus to alcohol in an unrecognized pregnancy than women who do not drink.

	Estimated annual average prevalence for levels of alcohol use		
	Nonuse[a] %[d]	Non-heavy use[b] %	Heavier use[c] %
Overall	**39.8**	**56.0**	**4.1**
Age			
18–24	46.6	48.2	5.1
25–34	37.7	58.7	3.6
35–44	37.3	58.7	4.0
Race/ethnicity			
Non-Hispanic White	31.2	63.6	5.2
Non-White or Hispanic	56.2	41.8	2.1
Education			
Less than college education	51.5	45.0	3.5
Some college education or higher	32.0	63.4	4.6
Currently employed			
No	52.9	44.1	3.0
Yes	33.6	61.7	4.7
Married			
No	38.8	55.5	5.8
Yes	40.7	56.6	2.7
Serious psychological distress			
No	39.6	56.3	4.1
Yes	41.4	52.8	5.7

[a] Nonuse is defined as no drinks in the past year.
[b] Non-heavy use is defined as consuming no more than 7 drinks per week for women in the past year, on average.
[c] Heavier use is defined as consuming more than 7 drinks per week for women in the past year, on average.
[d] Rows may not total 100 percent due to rounding.

Source: James Tsai et al., "Alcohol Use and Serious Psychological Distress Among Women of Childbearing Age," *Addictive Behaviors*, vol. 34, 2009.

49

- Fetal alcohol spectrum disorders are **100 percent** preventable and **100 percent** incurable.

- According to results from the 2009 National Survey on Drug Use and Health, which were published in 2010, **10 percent** of pregnant women aged 15 to 44 reported current alcohol use, **4.4 percent** reported binge drinking, and **0.8 percent** reported heavy drinking.

- The 2009 report "Alcohol Use Among Pregnant and Nonpregnant Women of Childbearing Age," published by the Centers for Disease Control and Prevention, shows an annual percentage of any alcohol use among pregnant women as **12.2 percent** when averaged over a recent 14-year time span.

- In a 2008 report in the journal *Alcoholism: Clinical and Experimental Research*, St. Louis University researchers revealed data that showed pregnant white women averaged nearly **80 percent** fewer drinks per month than nonpregnant white women, and about **85 percent** fewer binge drinking occasions. Pregnant black women averaged about **58 percent** fewer drinks per month than nonpregnant black women and **64 percent** fewer binge occasions.

- Data gleaned from the Canadian Community Health Survey and Canadian birth and population statistics suggest that **37 percent** of pregnant Canadian residents binge drink (5 or more drinks at one time) on multiple occasions during their pregnancies and that an additional **42 percent** drink 1 to 4 drinks on occasion during pregnancy.

What Are the Effects of Fetal Alcohol Disorders?

66Students with Fetal Alcohol Spectrum Disorders (FASD) have special learning needs and a wide range of behavioral challenges.99

—National Organization on Fetal Alcohol Syndrome.

66No two people with an FASD are exactly alike.99

—Centers for Disease Control and Prevention.

Withdrawal from Fetal Alcohol Exposure

Exposure to alcohol before birth not only puts a child at risk for fetal alcohol disorders, but it also puts an infant at risk of being born with neonatal withdrawal syndrome. Alcohol is a depressant and slows down the functioning of the brain and other parts of the central nervous system. If a fetus is exposed to alcohol regularly, it responds by producing greater-than-usual amounts of natural stimulants to counteract the depressant effects of alcohol. When an alcohol-exposed infant is born, its brain still produces extra stimulants even though the alcohol is no longer present, which results in the effects of withdrawal.

Withdrawal from alcohol exposure during prenatal development includes agitation, crying, sleeplessness, gastrointestinal upset, sneezing, and hiccupping. Infants may also have seizures, appear rigid, pull away and arch the back when held, and move about wildly. These previously alcohol-exposed infants may try to soothe themselves by sucking—as infants usually do—but they may have a poor sucking ability due to a fetal alcohol disorder. Thus, these infants cannot self-soothe. If their sucking ability is good, however, they may drink too much while frantically sucking on a bottle and then spit up. The effects of neonatal withdrawal syndrome usually subside within a few days to a week.

Effects on Infants and Toddlers

The National Organization on Fetal Alcohol Syndrome lists many effects of fetal alcohol spectrum disorders on infants, including low birth weight; irritability; sensitivity to light, noises, and touch; poor sucking; slow development; poor sleep-wake cycles; and increased ear infections. Sherry Martz shares a few memories about her first year with her adopted son that reveal some of these effects: "He wanted to be carried around as an infant, but not cradled in our arms. He hated to have his clothes or diaper changed and would scream every time. He is still colicky. . . . He would take an hour or longer to take just one bottle at night. About the time I got him back to sleep it was time for him to eat again."[11]

> " Exposure to alcohol before birth not only puts a child at risk for fetal alcohol disorders, but it also puts an infant at risk of being born with neonatal withdrawal syndrome. "

Infants with a fetal alcohol disorder may also be born with microcephaly, a condition that results in a significantly smaller-than-average size head. Some children with microcephaly develop normally and have normal intellectual function. However, others experience developmental delays, problems with coordination and balance, mental retardation, hyperactivity, dwarfism, facial distortions, and seizures.

As the FASD infant develops into a toddler, beginning at about age one, a poor memory and developmental delays may start to become evident if they have not already. The "terrible twos," which are often challenging for parents, may be even more challenging if a child has been exposed to alcohol during prenatal development. The toddler with a fetal alcohol disorder may be hyperactive, have no sense of boundaries, and be fearless. He or she also may become easily upset, startled, or distracted. Many toddlers with a fetal alcohol disorder have a short attention span. These disabilities result in a young child who may unexpectedly do things that are quite dangerous, such as running into the street even when cars are coming, and who may be a continual tornado of movement and sound while jumping from activity to activity.

School Performance

During the elementary school years, many learning challenges become evident in FASD children. According to the Substance Abuse and Mental Health Services Administration, these challenges include problems with processing what is seen, heard, and read. In addition, the FASD child may have difficulty remembering, paying attention, following directions and rules, understanding cause and effect, and organizing tasks and materials. For many children with a fetal alcohol disorder, math is the most difficult subject because they are unable to think and reason abstractly. Some children with a fetal alcohol disorder may have mental retardation as well.

Susan Rose, director of the Fetal Alcohol Support Network of New York City and Long Island, describes Kate, a teenager diagnosed with alcohol-related neurodevelopmental disorder. Before her diagnosis at age 17, the origin of Kate's problems was a mystery, and Kate was faltering. "School became increasingly frustrating because she was unable to think abstractly,"

> " One of the behavioral challenges of FASD children is that they are usually developmentally delayed, and their behaviors are like those of much younger children. "

says Rose. "She also kept losing and forgetting things. Other children were progressing in school, and Kate knew that she could not keep up with them."[12]

Like Kate, as the child with a fetal alcohol disorder progresses in school, he or she may have continual problems keeping up with the work.

In addition, FASD children may have developmental delays, which also serve to keep them behind their classmates. Thus, many FASD children develop low self-esteem. If these children are not diagnosed and helped, they cannot receive appropriate services and interventions to help pull them out of a downward spiral of negative educational outcomes.

Behavioral Challenges That Affect Learning

One of the behavioral challenges of FASD children is that they are usually developmentally delayed, and their behaviors are like those of much younger children. For example, a developmentally delayed FASD child who is 13 may have a developmental age of about 8. Thus, children with fetal alcohol disorders often act as if they were much younger than similar-aged peers.

Another of the behavioral challenges of FASD children is that their brains work in dysfunctional ways, so many of their behaviors are dysfunctional. For example, FASD children often have no impulse control, so they may disrupt class with inappropriate behavior like talking loudly when the teacher is talking. They may be overly physical because they do not understand personal space and boundaries, may not sit still because they need to move while learning, and may be jittery in class because they are experiencing sensory overload. In addition, FASD children may be late to class often because they cannot understand the abstract concept of time. Their organizational skills are often poor, so their work will likely be unorganized unless they receive assistance. And children with a fetal alcohol disorder often appear willfully not to do what the teacher asks, but actually they are just having trouble understanding what the teacher really wants them to do.

Social Interaction

The developmental immaturity of children with fetal alcohol disorders is evident not only in the classroom, but also in their social interactions. Although children with such disorders are generally outgoing, they are also hungry for attention and appear to others to be too talkative and intrusive. They do not understand social norms within a group and how to interact appropriately with others. For example, they often do not know how to "read" the facial expressions and body language of others, so they may not understand if someone feels insulted by something they did or said. They may take things without asking, interrupt others while they are talking, and use sarcasm at the wrong time or in the wrong context. Because of their social ineptness, children with fetal alcohol disorders have trouble establishing friendships and, as a result, often become socially isolated.

Daily Life Skills

Many daily life skills, such as getting dressed, making a sandwich, and using a fork and knife are difficult for individuals with FASD because they have problems with gross and fine motor skills. Gross motor skills, such as sitting upright, balancing, running, bike riding, and playing ball involve the larger muscles, such as those of the legs and arms. Fine motor skills, such as handwriting, picking up small objects, tying shoelaces, using scissors, and holding a cup by its handle, involve small muscles, such as those of the fingers.

Poor motor skills, eye-hand coordination, and body awareness not only hamper the ability of individuals with FASDs to accomplish daily tasks like taking a shower and washing their hair, but these disabilities also interfere with classroom interactions and day-to-day life. For example, FASD children move their

> " **Adults with fetal alcohol disorders usually require supervision around the clock so that they will not hurt themselves, unwittingly hurt others, or become the victim of abuse.** "

chairs a lot and often fall out of their chairs. They lean against furniture to help themselves remain upright, bump into people and furniture when trying to walk past, and apply too much force to a motion. Instead of tagging someone gently in a game, the FASD child may forcefully push; instead of holding someone's hand gently, he or she may squeeze it tightly—much too tightly.

Adults with Fetal Alcohol Disorders

Cara Hetland and Tom Robertson, in the Minnesota Public Radio multipart series *Fetal Alcohol Syndrome: The Invisible Disorder*, interviewed Hunter Sargent, a 31-year-old adult with fetal alcohol syndrome. Sargent lives in a subsidized apartment and has a personal care attendant who visits and works with him daily. Hetland and Robertson describe Sargent like this: "Sargent has no job and he can't drive a car. He gets a monthly Social Security check because he's considered mentally disabled. He has poor eyesight and poor balance. He says his math skills are limited to counting on his fingers. Like many adults with fetal alcohol syndrome, Hunter can't manage his own money."[13] Sargent explains that his impulsivity and poor money skills led him to develop huge bills when he was first on his own. He feels like he is constantly struggling to keep the effects of his fetal alcohol syndrome under control.

> **Over 90 percent of individuals with fetal alcohol disorders also have mental health problems.**

Most adults with fetal alcohol disorders are not able to live on their own like Sargent because of the many disabilities associated with such disorders. Most adults with fetal alcohol disorders have poor short-term memory, which means that they have difficulty remembering what they are doing moment to moment. In addition, individuals with such disorders often show poor judgment and have problems with impulse control. These disabilities create a situation in which individuals can easily compromise their safety or the safety of others. These disabilities also make it hard for adults with fetal alcohol disorders to get and keep a job.

Adults with fetal alcohol disorders usually require supervision around the clock so that they will not hurt themselves, unwittingly hurt others, or become the victim of abuse. Thus, FASD adults must live at home with their parents, in another homelike setting with foster parents or other caring individuals, or in a residential placement. Residential placement options include state institutions, community care facilities, and semi-independent living facilities. State institutions usually provide medical care, therapy, and daily living assistance. Community care facilities provide round-the-clock nonmedical care to children and adults who need supervision, protection, and assistance. Semi-independent living facilities are for adults only and provide less oversight. However, individuals admitted to semi-independent living facilities must exhibit basic adult living skills upon admission, and it is difficult for most individuals with fetal alcohol disorders to meet this requirement.

Common Secondary Disabilities

Individuals with a fetal alcohol disorder are born with primary disabilities. These disabilities are due directly to dysfunction of the brain and other parts of the central nervous system. Primary disabilities include poor memory, attention deficits, mental retardation, impulsivity, hyperactivity, volatile emotions, and difficulty with hearing, vision, abstract thinking, and cause and effect.

Individuals with fetal alcohol disorders are *not* born with secondary disabilities. These disabilities result from the primary disabilities as FASD individuals interact with their environments and with others. Secondary disabilities include mental health problems, a disrupted school experience (suspension, expulsion, or dropping out), trouble with the law, confinement (inpatient treatment for either mental health issues or drug treatment, or incarceration), inappropriate sexual behavior, and alcohol and drug problems.

The Substance Abuse and Mental Health Services Administration cites the work of psychologist Ann Streissguth, one of the researchers who undertook groundbreaking work on the original scientific identification and description of fetal alcohol syndrome in 1973, on secondary disabilities. Her research shows that over 90 percent of individuals with fetal alcohol disorders also have mental health problems. Over 40 percent are either suspended or expelled from school, or they drop out. An equivalent percentage gets into trouble with the law. About 45 percent exhibit inappropriate sexual behaviors, while 20 percent have problems with alcohol and other drugs. Well over 30 percent end up in institutions for mental health problems, drug and alcohol abuse, or breaking the law.

As the individual with fetal alcohol disorders experiences increasing problems with secondary disabilities, they may become viewed as beyond help. People are never beyond help, of course. But early diagnosis and intervention are crucial to help individuals with fetal alcohol disorders before their problems deepen and multiply.

What Are the Effects of Fetal Alcohol Disorders?

66 **People with FASDs who live in stable, non-abusive households or who do not become involved in youth violence are much less likely to develop secondary conditions than children who have been exposed to violence in their lives.** 99

—Centers for Disease Control and Prevention, "Fetal Alcohol Spectrum Disorders (FASDs)," August 19, 2009.
www.cdc.gov.

The Centers for Disease Control and Prevention is the nation's premier agency for health promotion and operates under the US Department of Health and Human Services.

66 **Results suggest that alcohol-exposed adolescents have substantial impairments in their abilities to solve problems in their everyday life, even in the absence of mental retardation.** 99

—Christie L. McGee et al., "Deficits in Social Problem Solving in Adolescents with Prenatal Exposure to Alcohol,"
American Journal of Drug and Alcohol Abuse, 2008.

The authors are clinical researchers in the Department of Psychology and at the Center for Behavioral Teratology, San Diego State University.

* Editor's Note: While the definition of a primary source can be narrowly or broadly defined, for the purposes of Compact Research, a primary source consists of: 1) results of original research presented by an organization or researcher; 2) eyewitness accounts of events, personal experience, or work experience; 3) first-person editorials offering pundits' opinions; 4) government officials presenting political plans and/or policies; 5) representatives of organizations presenting testimony or policy.

❝The child with an FASD has a hidden disability.❞

—Anne Hedelius, "The ABC's of Parenting a Child with an FASD," *Iceberg Newsletter*, September 2009. http://fasiceberg.org.

Hedelius is a licensed social worker and an adoptive mother of children with FASDs.

❝It is very common for people with FAS to not only lose their virginity early but to be very promiscuous as well.❞

—Jennifer Poss Taylor, *Forfeiting All Sanity: A Mother's Story of Raising a Child with Fetal Alcohol Syndrome*. Mustang, OK: Tate, 2010.

Taylor is an adoptive mother of a daughter with FAS.

❝Prenatal alcohol exposure is not strongly related to young adult substance use.❞

—Maternal Substance Abuse and Child Development Project, "Alcohol and Drug Use in Young Adults with Prenatal Alcohol Exposure," 2009. www.psychiatry.emory.edu.

The Maternal Substance Abuse and Child Development Project at Emory University in Atlanta, Georgia, works with children and adults affected by fetal alcohol disorders.

❝Current evidence of the effects of prenatal alcohol exposure on behaviour suggests that any postulated association between the two is complex.❞

—Gayle P. Dolan, David H. Stone, and Andrew H. Briggs, "Cognitive Effects: A Systematic Review of Continuous Performance Task Research in Children Prenatally Exposed to Alcohol," *Alcohol and Alcoholism*, December 7, 2009.

The authors are medical researchers at the University of Glasgow in the United Kingdom.

66 These data reveal that in general, children with mild FASD perform similarly to their peers in the classroom during both small group and large group activities with regard to behavior states/dimensions. 99

—Lesley B. Olswang, Liselotte Svensson, and Susan Astley, "Observation of Classroom Social Communication: Do Children with Fetal Alcohol Spectrum Disorders Spend Their Time Differently than Their Peers Developing Typically?" *Journal of Speech, Language, and Hearing Research*, August 12, 2010.

The authors are speech, language, and hearing clinical researchers. Olswang and Astley are at the University of Washington in Seattle and Svensson is at the Karolinska Institute in Stockholm, Sweden.

Facts and Illustrations

What Are the Effects of Fetal Alcohol Disorders?

- Results of a study published in the June 2010 issue of *Alcoholism: Clinical and Experimental Research* showed a high prevalence of epilepsy (**5.9 percent**) in individuals with fetal alcohol disorders compared with individuals who did not have such disorders (**0.6 percent**).

- The National Organization on Fetal Alcohol Syndrome notes that about **60 percent** of individuals with a fetal alcohol disorder find themselves in legal trouble at some point in their lives.

- In a 2010 article in the *Journal of Neuropsychiatric Disease and Treatment,* researchers noted that **94 percent** of individuals heavily exposed to alcohol in the womb are diagnosed with attention deficit hyperactivity disorder.

- Results of a study conducted by researchers at the National Institute of Environmental Health Sciences show that pregnant women who engaged in binge drinking in their first trimester are more than twice as likely as pregnant nondrinkers to give birth to infants with **cleft lip with or without cleft palate**, or **cleft palate** alone.

- The National Organization on Fetal Alcohol Syndrome notes that **35 percent** of individuals with fetal alcohol disorders who are over the age of 12 had been imprisoned at some point in their lives.

Health Conditions Common to Fetal Alcohol Disorders

Children with fetal alcohol syndrome disorders (FASDs) have a higher prevalence of certain other health conditions than children not affected by FASDs. A study comparing 89 children with FASDs to those without (a control group of 92) found that sleep disorders and attention deficit hyperactivity disorder are among the most common health conditions found in children with fetal alcohol disorders.

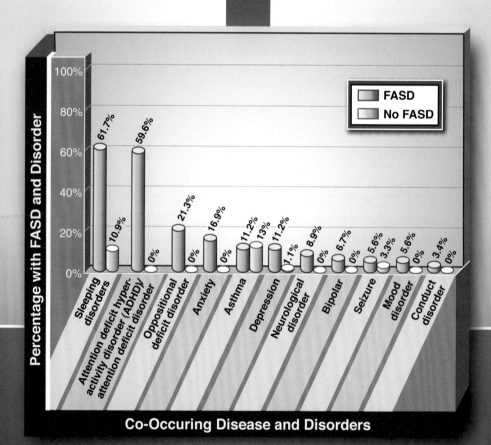

Percentage with FASD and Disorder

Legend: FASD, No FASD

- Sleeping disorders: 61.7%, 10.9%
- Attention deficit hyperactivity disorder (ADHD)/attention deficit disorder: 59.6%, 0%
- Oppositional deficit disorder: 21.3%, 0%
- Anxiety: 16.9%, 0%
- Asthma: 11.2%, 13%
- Depression: 11.2%, 1.1%
- Neurological disorder: 8.9%, 0%
- Bipolar: 6.7%, 0%
- Seizure: 5.6%, 3.3%
- Mood disorder: 5.6%, 0%
- Conduct disorder: 3.4%, 0%

Co-Occuring Disease and Disorders

Source: C.R. Green et al., "Executive Function Deficits in Children with Fetal Alcohol Spectrum Disorders (FASD) Measured Using the Cambridge Neuropsychological Tests Automated Battery (CANTAB)," *The Journal of Child Psychology and Psychiatry*, June 2009.

Characteristics of Adults with Fetal Alcohol Disorders

As part of a study of adults with fetal alcohol disorders, researchers compiled a list of the characteristics of study participants. The most common characteristics included vulnerability to manipulation, being diagnosed with some type of mental health problem, and having experienced some form of violence.

Characteristics	Percent
Under 20 years old	37%
Living with a caregiver	69%
Had at least one child	26%
Of those who had a child or children, still involved in parenting	56%
Diagnosed before age 6	34%
Vulnerable to manipulation	92%
Ever experienced violence	87%
Verbal	81%
Physical	69%
Sexual	55%
Receives support living services	26%
Intelligence quotient ≤ 70	34%
Functional assessment	
Minimal level of care required	7%
Low level of care required	13%
Moderate level of care required	37%
High level of care required	44%
Secondary disability	
Mental health diagnosis	92%
Disruptive school experience	61%
Trouble with the law	45%
Displays sexually inappropriate behavior	45%
Ever confined to a hospital or prison	32%
Ever had an alcohol or drug problem	22%

Source: Erica Clark et al., "Caregiver Perceptions of the Community Integration of Adults with Fetal Alcohol Spectrum Disorder in British Columbia," *Journal of Applied Research in Intellectual Disabilities*, September 1, 2008.

Prevalence of Epilepsy and Seizures in Populations with FASDs

The prevalence of epilepsy—a seizure disorder—is 0.6 percent in the general population. It is 10 times that, or nearly 6 percent, in populations of individuals with fetal alcohol disorders. Individuals with one form of FASD, alcohol-related neurodevelopmental disorder, make up the the FASD group with the highest prevalence of epilepsy. Those with fetal alcohol syndrome make up the group with the highest prevalence of all seizures.

Epilepsy and Seizures in FASD Population

FASD diagnosis	No seizures	≥1 seizure episode(s)	Epilepsy	All seizures
FAS	80%	20%	0%	20%
pFAS	85.9%	9.9%	4.2%	14.1%
ARND	81.7%	11.8%	6.5%	18.23%
Overall	82.3%	11.8%	5.9%	17.7%

Source: Stephanie H. Bell, "The Remarkably High Prevalence of Epilepsy and Seizure History in Fetal Alcohol Spectrum Disorders," *Alcoholism: Clinical and Experimental Research*, June 2010.

- Results of research conducted by Ann Streissguth and colleagues found that **50 percent** of adults with fetal alcohol disorders were clinically depressed.

- The average IQ of children with fetal alcohol syndrome is **68**, which is considered **mild mental retardation**.

- A Swedish study found that **one-quarter** of all eight- and nine-year-old children who had alcoholic birth mothers attended schools for those with intellectual disabilities.

- Researchers from the University of Washington Fetal Alcohol Syndrome Diagnostic and Prevention Network determined that nearly half (**48 percent**) of children with a fetal alcohol disorder needed extensive or frequent support to succeed.

- Exposure to alcohol before birth has been associated with more than **60 disease conditions, birth defects, and disabilities.**

- The Fetal Alcohol Disorders Society reports that **10 to 15 percent** of children are likely affected by prenatal alcohol exposure to the extent that they need special education services.

- The National Organization on Fetal Alcohol Syndrome notes that the annual cost to Americans for fetal alcohol syndrome, the least common and most severe fetal alcohol disorder, is estimated at **$5.4 billion.**

- The estimated lifetime cost for one individual with fetal alcohol syndrome is **$2 million.**

How Can Individuals with Fetal Alcohol Disorders Be Helped?

❝Structure is the 'glue' that makes the world make sense for a student with FAS. If this glue is taken away, the walls fall down! A student with FAS achieves and is successful because their world provides the appropriate structure as a permanent foundation.❞

—Deb Evensen and Jan Lutke, Fasalaska Project FACTS (Fetal Alcohol Consultation and Training Services).

❝A child who is diagnosed at a young age can be placed in appropriate educational classes and get the social services needed to help the child and his or her family.❞

—National Center on Birth Defects and Developmental Disabilities, Centers for Disease Control and Prevention.

There are many techniques, strategies, and interventions for helping a child with a fetal alcohol disorder. Jeanne, the mother of a teenage son with such a disorder, knows most of them but still acknowledges the enormous challenges of nurturing an FASD child. Jeanne says that "raising a child with FASD is a lot like climbing an endless mountain. . . . You struggle for answers, look for techniques, beg for help and yet, the rocks keep falling and storms keep raging. . . . You retreat to base camp and hope that one day you will be able to catch a glimpse of the top of the mountain. Many don't realize that when families struggle with FASD, it is 24/7, forever."[14]

Early Intervention Treatment

Treatment for fetal alcohol disorders can start at birth. Early intervention treatment helps developmentally delayed babies and toddlers through age two learn to do the things infants and toddlers usually do during this phase of their lives. This includes talking, listening, thinking, learning, solving problems, walking, playing, eating, and interacting with others. Although FASDs are permanent disabilities—they cannot be cured—treatment can help the child with such a disorder improve his or her development. The earlier in life treatment is begun, the better are the chances of improvement.

Early intervention treatment for developmentally delayed and otherwise disabled infants and toddlers is provided for in the Individuals with Disabilities Education Act. This act was originally passed in 1975, and the provision for infants and toddlers was added in 1986.

The first step to early intervention treatment is an evaluation by a team of education specialists. Those eligible are then assessed to determine the services they need. The family's needs are assessed as well. These assessments result in an Individualized Family Service Plan, which includes such interventions as family training, speech therapy, hearing impairment services, physical therapy, and psychological services.

Interventions for Preschool and School-Age Children

Early intervention services end when a child turns three years old, but children who need continuing help are transitioned to special education services. These services focus on the child alone and are directed by the school system. Parents are involved in meetings regarding the child and his or her progress, but decisions about treatment and interventions ultimately rest with the education professionals.

A team of school professionals develop the child's Individualized Education Plan. The plan lists the programs, supplemental aids, program modifications, and accommodations that will be made for the child and the amount of time the child will spend in the special education classroom and the regular classroom. It also lists individuals who will be involved in the child's education and the role each person will play. Goals are listed as well. Periodically, progress toward the goals is evaluated, and the plan may be revised by the team. As the child moves through preschool and into elementary school, he or she is reevaluated every three years to determine whether special education services are still needed.

Successful Strategies at School

The National Organization on Fetal Alcohol Syndrome lists common areas of concern in the classroom and strategies that help accommodate these concerns. Students with fetal alcohol disorders have difficulty with attention, organizational skills, abstract thinking, and coping mechanisms, among other disabilities. In order to help students and facilitate learning, teachers can structure the classroom, their teaching strategies, and their approach to behavior in ways that accommodate these problems. Teachers who work with students diagnosed with a fetal alcohol disorder are usually trained in an array of teaching strategies that help those students.

> " Early intervention treatment for developmentally delayed and otherwise disabled infants and toddlers is provided for in the Individuals with Disabilities Education Act. This act was originally passed in 1975. "

There are some overarching themes that can be seen among the more specific strategies teachers use with FASD children. For example, individuals with a fetal alcohol disorder experience sensory overload very easily. Thus, the classroom environment is kept as quiet and serene as possible, with less visual stimulation than the usual classroom. In addition, consistency, repetition, and routine are key attributes to the learning situation. Consistency is important because the child with a fetal alcohol disorder has problems generalizing from one situation to another. Doing things the same way and giving directions the same way—using the same key phrases, for instance—

help understanding. Repetition aids short-term memory, as does giving directions one step at a time. A stable routine decreases the anxiety of those with fetal alcohol disorders and helps them anticipate what will happen next. Visual aids—using objects and images in teaching—help make abstract concepts concrete. In addition, supervision of children with such disorders is constant

> " **Socially, FASD children often play well with younger children, since the child with the disorder is developmentally delayed.** "

because they are developmentally much younger than their chronological age, have poor impulse control, and have difficulty understanding cause and effect. Therefore, they can become involved in troublesome, disruptive, and unsafe situations quickly.

Successful Strategies at Home

Many of the strategies that are successful at school work at home as well. For example, a simple and quiet home environment, clear routines, structure, and repetition all help the child with a fetal alcohol disorder. Routines, structure, and repetition matter because having a fetal alcohol disorder has been described as feeling like someone is continually rearranging your kitchen or your closet, and you never know where anything is. Dressing is difficult because you cannot find your clothes. Cooking is impossible when the food is no longer in the refrigerator. Providing a high level of routine and structure helps keep life in order for the child who feels internal disorder.

Socially, FASD children often play well with younger children, since the child with the disorder is developmentally delayed. They also enjoy short, structured activities, since the attention span of the FASD child is short. And if the child with a fetal alcohol disorder has a tantrum, he or she often calms down when removed from the situation and is given a warm bath or is rocked. When asked, professional counselors, educators, or psychologists often help educate parents in specific techniques to help them manage the particular behaviors or problems that their child presents.

Behavior and Education Therapy

Various therapies have been shown to help some children with FASDs: friendship training, specialized math tutoring, executive functioning training, parent-child interaction therapy, and parenting and behavior management training. A person trained in the therapy works with the child, or with the child and parents, to help the child overcome specific difficulties or strengthen certain positive behaviors.

Friendship training occurs over a three-month period, with one group session per week conducted by clinicians. In the sessions children learn social skills and appropriate ways to behave with others in particular situations. Parents have sessions as well to learn what their children are learning so that they can support the process.

Parents also develop skills to help their children in parent-child interaction therapy and in parenting and behavior management training.

> **Math tutoring helps children with FASDs develop their working memory—the ability to hold something in the mind, such as numbers, while the mind works with the numbers to solve a problem.**

In parent-child interaction therapy, parents are taught how to use specific techniques while playing with their child that will help strengthen the parent-child relationship, decrease negative behaviors in the child, and increase positive behaviors. In the parenting and behavior management training, parents learn how to manage behavioral problems in their children by using techniques such as consistent and stable routines, positive reinforcement, and a simplified environment.

Both specialized math tutoring and executive functioning training help children with fetal alcohol disorders improve their cognitive skills. Executive functioning refers to higher-level cognitive operations that control and manage other cognitive functions. Some executive functions include remembering, writing, starting and finishing work, solving problems, and controlling emotions. For example, in planning a trip, it is the executive functioning that helps an individual remember, plan, and organize so that all of the factors involved will be ready and in place at the right time. Executive functioning training uses a variety of techniques to help children develop executive function. For example, cognitive behavioral interventions help children to think about their thinking before they behave impulsively, and to mentally talk themselves through an appropriate response or action.

> **Therapists help those with fetal alcohol disorders develop strategies to cope with daily life situations, build and maintain healthy relationships, and remain safe.**

Prenatal alcohol exposure often affects parts of the brain that are involved in math skills. Math tutoring helps children with FASDs develop their working memory—the ability to hold something in the mind, such as numbers, while the mind works with the numbers to solve a problem. Math tutoring for children with such disorders also focuses on using objects a child can touch and manipulate, not only to teach the math concepts in a more concrete manner but also to help develop visual-spatial relationships.

Drug Therapy

No medications are approved specifically for use in individuals with fetal alcohol disorders. Some medications, however, are used to treat the symptoms of these disorders, because they help restore a chemical balance in the brain. The Centers for Disease Control and Prevention describes four types of medications that are currently used: stimulants, neuroleptics, antidepressants, and antianxiety drugs.

Stimulants, such as Ritalin, Adderall, and Dexedrine are used to treat a variety of conditions found in FASD children, such as attention deficit disorder, hyperactivity, and poor impulse control. Although it would seem that stimulants would intensify these problems, they actually help to settle down hyperactivity, improve impulse control, and increase focus for many individuals by increasing the levels of chemicals in the brain that transmit nerve signals. Neuroleptic drugs, also called antipsychotics, help transmit nerve signals in the brain as well, thereby improving behavior in children with fetal alcohol disorders. Antidepressants, such as Elavil and Cymbalta, help individuals with these disorders who may be irritable, aggressive, or sad, or who have problems with sleeping, socialization, or negativity. In addition, antianxiety drugs, also known as tranquilizers, help some children with fetal alcohol disorders feel less distressed.

Counseling and Psychotherapy

Counseling and psychotherapy is the treatment of mental and emotional problems by licensed practitioners who talk to patients and work through problems verbally. Therapists help those with fetal alcohol disorders develop strategies to cope with daily life situations, build and maintain healthy relationships, and remain safe. They also help their patients figure out their needs and how to satisfy them, such as finding housing or financial support. They also counsel them on sexual matters, to help avoid pregnancy and sexually transmitted infections. In addition, counselors and psychotherapists who work with FASD patients determine whether the patients have medical or psychiatric disorders or substance abuse problems that need the care of specialists.

Social Services and Support Networks

Social services are welfare activities for individuals or families that are carried out in the home by trained personnel. According to researchers at St. Louis University, there are no social service programs in the United States designed specifically to help children and young adults with fetal alcohol disorders. To fill this need, researchers from St. Louis University along with colleagues from the University of California–Los Angeles have developed a social service program for older children and adults with FASDs called Partners for Success. In this program, individuals with such a disorder are each paired with a mentor who models appropriate behavior and teaches daily living skills in biweekly home sessions. According to the researchers, the techniques they are using are based on well-established research, but their efforts are still a focus of study. The researchers are hopeful that the Partners for Success approach will be a highly effective way to support individuals with fetal alcohol disorders.

Support networks include groups of people and organizations that provide help, information, and encouragement to FASD individuals, their families, and other persons who work with those afflicted with such disorders. There are international, national, state, and local organizations.

Sixteen-year-old Anique, a tenth grader with fetal alcohol syndrome, sums up how those with FASDs can be best helped: "Don't let people punish us for mistakes or freaking out because we don't do it on purpose. We do not forget or lie or show up late at an appointment on purpose, either. You need to make sure we have a good home where people understand us and accept us."[15] Although various strategies, programs, and interventions work to help those with a fetal alcohol disorder maneuver their way through life, as Anique suggests, understanding and acceptance are the factors that matter the most.

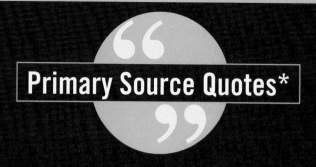

How Can Individuals with Fetal Alcohol Disorders Be Helped?

Primary Source Quotes

"While teaching young adults with Fetal Alcohol Spectrum Disorder [FASD] is challenging, those working with FASD students know there is great potential for those students to lead meaningful lives."

—Kelly Edmonds and Susan Crichton, "Finding Ways to Teach Students with FASD: A Research Study," *International Journal of Special Education*, 2008.

Edmonds and Crichton are educational researchers who conducted this study while at the University of Calgary in Alberta, Canada. Crichton is currently a faculty member at the University of Calgary.

"Children with FASDs can be more sensitive than other children to disruptions, changes in lifestyle or routines, and harmful relationships."

—National Center on Birth Defects and Developmental Disabilities, "Fetal Alcohol Spectrum Disorders (FASDs)," Centers for Disease Control and Prevention, August 19, 2009. www.cdc.gov.

The National Center on Birth Defects and Developmental Disabilities is a division of the Centers for Disease Control and Prevention, the nation's premier health protection office.

* Editor's Note: While the definition of a primary source can be narrowly or broadly defined, for the purposes of Compact Research, a primary source consists of: 1) results of original research presented by an organization or researcher; 2) eyewitness accounts of events, personal experience, or work experience; 3) first-person editorials offering pundits' opinions; 4) government officials presenting political plans and/or policies; 5) representatives of organizations presenting testimony or policy.

66 **Although FAS was identified in the U.S. over 35 years ago, the development, evaluation, and dissemination of evidence-based interventions for individuals with FASDs have lagged behind significantly.** 99

—Blair Paley and Mary J. O'Connor, "Intervention for Individuals with Fetal Alcohol Spectrum Disorders: Treatment Approaches and Case Management," *Developmental Disabilities Research Reviews*, 2009.

Paley and O'Connor are researchers at the Semel Institute for Neuroscience and Human Behavior at the University of California–Los Angeles.

66 **Just as we accommodate physically handicapped people with wheelchairs and ramps, blind people with seeing-eye dogs, and the hard-of-hearing with hearing aids, we also need to make environmental accommodations for those with brain differences.** 99

—Minnesota Organization on Fetal Alcohol Syndrome, "Reframing the Challenges of Fetal Alcohol Spectrum Disorders," February 2010. www.mofas.org.

The Minnesota Organization on Fetal Alcohol Syndrome is a nonprofit organization that has been providing training, information, resources, and support on fetal alcohol disorders to Minnesota residents since 1998.

66 **If you keep in mind that children with FASD have a hard time communicating, their inappropriate behavior no longer seems malicious or irrational.** 99

—Pregnancy and Alcohol.org, "Fetal Alcohol Spectrum Disorders," 2010. http://pregnancyandalcohol.org.

Pregnancy and Alcohol.org is a nonprofit website run by the Wisconsin Treatment Outreach Project and the Family Empowerment Network of the University of Wisconsin School of Medicine and Public Health, Department of Family Medicine.

**"Over the years we parents have learned that aware-
ness of the behaviors that are the result of neurological damage can make the difference between success
for our children and frustrating failure."**

—Jocie DeVries with Delinda McCann, "DSM-V: Making the Case for an FASD Behavioral Phenotype," *Iceberg Newsletter*, March 2010.

DeVries is an adoptive parent of a son with a fetal alcohol disorder and the executive director of the nonprofit FAS Family Resource Institute.

....

**"Children who receive special education geared to-
wards their specific needs and learning style are more
likely to reach their full potential."**

—National Center on Birth Defects and Developmental Disabilities, "Fetal Alcohol Spectrum Disorders (FASDs)," Centers for Disease Control and Prevention, August 19, 2009. www.cdc.gov.

The National Center on Birth Defects and Developmental Disabilities is a division of the Centers for Disease Control and Prevention, the nation's premier
health protection office.

....

**"Lying is very common with almost all children with
FAS. They lie about anything and everything. It is their
way of having control on their uncontrollable lives."**

—Jennifer Poss Taylor, *Forfeiting All Sanity: A Mother's Story of Raising a Child with Fetal Alcohol Syndrome*. Mustang, OK: Tate, 2010.

Taylor is an adoptive mother of a daughter with fetal alcohol syndrome.

....

Facts and Illustrations

How Can Individuals with Fetal Alcohol Disorders Be Helped?

- A survey of pediatricians reported in the journal *Pediatrics* revealed that only **34 percent** felt equipped to supervise the treatment of children with a fetal alcohol disorder.

- In a random-sample survey of psychologists' knowledge about the diagnosis, treatment, and prevention of fetal alcohol disorders, **39 percent** responded that they were extremely unprepared to identify children with fetal alcohol syndrome or other alcohol-related disorders, **26 percent** said they were somewhat unprepared, and **26 percent** said they were somewhat prepared. Less than **4 percent** felt very prepared.

- According to the National Dissemination Center for Children with Disabilities, more than **6 million** children with disabilities receive special education programs and services each year in our nation's schools.

- Results of a study of adults with a fetal alcohol disorder, conducted by University of Washington researchers, revealed that **50 percent** had difficulty finding a job and **60 percent** had difficulty keeping a job. Only **18 percent** successfully lived on their own, while about **80 percent** had problems managing money and making decisions.

- Results of research conducted by Ann Streissguth and colleagues found that **58 percent** of adolescents with fetal alcohol disorders had trouble getting along with peers and **48 percent** had engaged in inappropriate sexual behavior.

Medications Can Help Children with FASDs

Children with FASDs often have other problems, such as sleeping disorders, attention-deficit/hyperactivity disorder, anxiety, and depression. Stimulants, antipsychotics, antidepressants, and other medications help to manage these conditions. The table shows the percentage of children with FASDs who were prescribed certain medications.

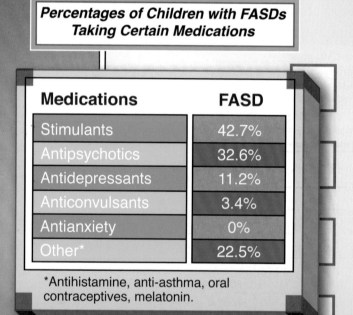

Percentages of Children with FASDs Taking Certain Medications

Medications	FASD
Stimulants	42.7%
Antipsychotics	32.6%
Antidepressants	11.2%
Anticonvulsants	3.4%
Antianxiety	0%
Other*	22.5%

*Antihistamine, anti-asthma, oral contraceptives, melatonin.

Note: Percentages add up to more than 100 percent because some children are taking more than one type of medication.

Source: C.R. Green et al., "Executive Function Deficits in Children with Fetal Alcohol Spectrum Disorders (FASD) Measured Using the Cambridge Neuropsychological Tests Automated Battery (CANTAB)," *The Journal of Child Psychology and Psychiatry*, June 2009.

- Data from the Child Psychiatric Inpatient Service at the University of California–Los Angeles show that children with fetal alcohol disorders are often prescribed a greater number of **psychiatric medications** simultaneously than are children without such disorders.

Families Helping Children with Fetal Alcohol Disorders

Researchers developing interventions to help children with fetal alcohol disorders interviewed their families to determine their unmet needs in caring for their FASD children. The quality of the home environment is important to the development of children with FASDs. However, parenting a child with an FASD can be extremely challenging, so meeting the needs of those caring and living with children with FASDs is important to both the health of the family and the child.

Caring for Children with Fetal Alcohol Spectrum Disorders

Percentage Indicating Need Is Unmet	Type of Family Need
69.2%	Discuss feelings about my child with someone who has gone through the same experience.
61.7%	Have help in preparing for the worst.
60.8%	Have enough resources for myself or the family.
58.8%	Have help in remaining hopeful about my child's future.
58%	Get a break from my problems and responsibilities.
52.9%	Have complete information on my child's thinking problems.
55.8%	Be reassured that it is usual to have negative feelings about changes in my child's behavior.
51%	Be shown what to do when my child is upset or acting strange.
48.1%	Be told why my child acts in ways that are different, difficult, or strange.
47.1%	Have different professionals agree on the best way to help my child.
47.1%	Pay attention to my own needs.

Source: Heather Carmichael Olson et al., "'Family Matters': Fetal Alcohol Spectrum Disorders and the Family," *Developmental Disabilities*, August 1, 2009.

Key People and Advocacy Groups

American Association of People with Disabilities: America's largest cross-disability membership organization, the American Association of People with Disabilities is an advocacy group for implementing the goals of the Americans with Disabilities Act.

Bonnie Buxton and Brian Philcox: Bonnie Buxton is a Canadian journalist who wrote *Damaged Angels: A Mother Discovers the Terrible Cost of Alcohol in Pregnancy*, published in 2004. The book is considered a significant contribution to the understanding of fetal alcohol disorders and chronicles Buxton and her husband, Brian Philcox's, many years of trying to determine what was wrong with their adopted daughter Colette.

Michael Dorris: The late Michael Dorris was the author of *The Broken Cord*, which was published in 1989 and influenced Congress to enact legislation to put warning labels on alcoholic beverage bottles citing the dangers of drinking alcohol during pregnancy. His book is based on raising his adopted Native American son.

Family Empowerment Network, University of Wisconsin School of Medicine and Public Health: The Family Empowerment Network is a support organization for parents, educational professionals, and health-care practitioners who deal with individuals with fetal alcohol disorders. The network provides information, training, and lists of resources, and its primary goal is to empower families affected by fetal alcohol disorders.

The FAS Family Resource Institute: The nonprofit FAS Family Resource Institute works to identify, understand, and care for individuals with fetal alcohol disorders and their families. They provide training, workshops, publications, assistance, referrals, and support.

FASlink Fetal Alcohol Disorders Society: FASlink was founded by Bruce Ritchie, the father of a son with fetal alcohol syndrome. FASlink is a primary Canadian resource on fetal alcohol disorders, providing information, support, and advocacy for those involved with individuals with these disorders.

FASworld: Founded by FASD advocates Bonnie Buxton and Brian Philcox, FASworld provides online and telephone counseling to those involved with fetal alcohol disorders. This Canada-based nonprofit organization works to reduce the incidence of these disorders through its public awareness programs, lectures, and workshops.

Kenneth Lyons Jones and David Smith: Kenneth Lyons Jones, pediatrician and birth defects researcher, is the chief of the Division of Dysmorphology/Teratology in the Department of Pediatrics at the University of California–San Diego. Jones and pediatrician David Smith were the first to identify and name fetal alcohol syndrome. Smith passed away in 1981; Jones recently received a lifetime achievement award in genetics from the March of Dimes.

Teresa Kellerman: An adoptive parent of a son with fetal alcohol syndrome, Teresa Kellerman is the director of the FAS Community Resource Center in Tucson, Arizona. For about 20 years, Kellerman has conducted training sessions and workshops and provided support and information for families on fetal alcohol disorders.

Ann Streissguth: Streissguth is professor emerita in the Department of Psychiatry and Behavioral Sciences at the University of Washington (UW) School of Medicine. She worked with David Smith and Kenneth Lyons Jones on the first clinical diagnoses of fetal alcohol syndrome in 1973 and went on to establish the Fetal Alcohol and Drug Unit at the UW School of Medicine.

Chronology

1726

England's College of Physicians recognizes gin as a cause of childhood disorders, increased stillbirth, and infant mortality after restrictions on distilling are lifted and the country experiences a gin "epidemic."

1899

William Sullivan, in one of the earliest thorough descriptions of fetal alcohol syndrome, finds higher rates of stillbirth and infant mortality among children of alcoholic mothers than children of nonalcoholic mothers.

1933

Prohibition ends in the United States, after which research on the effects of prenatal alcohol exposure slowly begins again.

1700   1800   1900   1930   1980

1834

During the temperance movement, a committee on drunkenness reports to the British House of Commons that infants of alcoholic mothers look starved and shriveled.

1967

Alexandre LeMache reports to the French Academy of Medicine his observations of hundreds of children born to alcoholic mothers over 37 years. This report marks the beginning of modern scientific research into the effects of fetal alcohol exposure on child development.

1973

Kenneth Lyons Jones and David Smith coin the diagnostic term "fetal alcohol syndrome" and develop its clinical description.

1920

Prohibition begins in the United States, contributing to a near halt on research on the effects of prenatal alcohol exposure.

1974

The National Institute on Alcohol Abuse and Alcoholism begins awarding grants for research projects on fetal alcohol syndrome.

1980
The Fetal Alcohol Study Group of the Research Society on Alcoholism standardizes the criteria for defining fetal alcohol syndrome and proposes the term "fetal alcohol effects," or FAE, to describe children who have some but not all features of the disorder.

2010
Ultrasound is used to help identify brain abnormalities during prenatal development so that early intervention services can be provided at birth.

1996
The Institute of Medicine defines and names diagnostic categories for prenatal alcohol-attributed effects in children: fetal alcohol syndrome, partial fetal alcohol syndrome, alcohol-related birth defects, and alcohol-related neurodevelopmental disorders.

1989
A new law requires all bottles of alcohol-containing beverages be labeled with a warning about the risks of drinking alcohol while pregnant.

1980   **1995**   **2010**

1994
Edward P. Riley and colleagues publish the first study that used magnetic resonance imaging on the brains of FASD children to show which areas of the central nervous system are affected by prenatal alcohol exposure.

2005
The US Surgeon General releases an advisory on drinking alcohol during pregnancy, urging women who are pregnant or who may become pregnant to refrain from drinking.

1981
The US Surgeon General advises women not to drink alcohol when pregnant because of alcohol's detrimental effects on the fetus.

2000
Researchers from the Fetal Alcohol and Drug Unit at the University of Washington School of Medicine in Seattle propose the phrase "fetal alcohol spectrum disorders," or FASDs, be used to describe the full range of conditions that result from prenatal alcohol exposure.

Related Organizations

American Academy of Pediatrics

141 Northwest Point Blvd.
Elk Grove Village, IL 60007-1098
phone: (847) 434-4000 • fax: (847) 434-8000
website: www.aap.org

The American Academy of Pediatrics is an organization dedicated to the health care, well-being, safety, and nurturing of children. The organization provides not only general information on child health and development but also information on specific conditions such as fetal alcohol spectrum disorders.

Collaborative Initiative on Fetal Alcohol Spectrum Disorders

Center for Behavioral Teratology
Department of Psychology
San Diego State University
6330 Alvarado Ct., Suite 100
San Diego, CA 92120
phone: (619) 594-4566 • fax: (619) 594-1895
e-mail: eriley@mail.sdsu.edu • website: www.cifasd.org

The Collaborative Initiative on Fetal Alcohol Spectrum Disorders is a worldwide consortium of researchers at 15 participating university sites, coordinated by the Center for Behavioral Teratology at San Diego State University. The researchers work together to develop effective interventions and treatment approaches for fetal alcohol disorders.

FAS Diagnostic and Prevention Network

Center on Human Development & Disability
University of Washington
Box 357920
Seattle, WA 98195
phone: (206) 543-7701
e-mail: fasdpn@uw.edu • website: http://depts.washington.edu/fasdpn

This network is a system of five medical clinics in Washington State linked through the Center on Human Development and Disability at the University of Washington in Seattle. Its mission is the prevention of fetal alcohol syndrome through screening, diagnosis, intervention, training, education, and research.

FASSTAR Enterprises

7725 E. 33rd St.
Tucson, AZ 85710
phone: (520) 296-9172
e-mail: tkellerman@cox.net • website: http://fasstar.com

The president of FASSTAR Enterprises is Teresa Kellerman, an adoptive mother of a young man with fetal alcohol syndrome. She is also director of the FAS Community Resource Center in Tucson, AZ. Kellerman offers training and workshops in fetal alcohol disorders and provides information on these disorders on the above website.

Fetal Alcohol and Drug Unit

Department of Psychiatry and Behavioral Sciences
University of Washington School of Medicine
180 Nickerson St., Suite 309
Seattle, WA 98109
phone (206) 543-7155 • fax (206) 685-2903
website: http://depts.washington.edu/fadu

The Fetal Alcohol and Drug Unit conducts research, disseminates information, and consults with individuals and families on fetal alcohol syndrome, other fetal alcohol disorders, and the effects of other drugs on fetal development.

March of Dimes

1275 Mamaroneck Ave.
White Plains, NY 10605
phone: (914) 997-4488
website: www.marchofdimes.com

Improving the health of babies is the primary mission of the March of Dimes. The organization focuses on preventing birth defects, premature births, low birth weight, and infant deaths via research, community service, and education.

Maternal Substance Abuse and Child Development Project

Emory University West
1256 Briarcliff Rd., Room-323 West
Atlanta, GA 30306
phone: (404) 712-9800 • fax: (404) 712-9809
website: www.psychiatry.emory.edu/PROGRAMS/GADrug

Originally known as the Fetal Alcohol Syndrome Screening Project, this group developed a screening tool that identifies children and adolescents with effects from prenatal alcohol exposure. The organization continues to work with children and adults affected by fetal alcohol disorders, focusing on the long-term effects of alcohol exposure in the womb.

National Center on Birth Defects and Developmental Disabilities

Centers for Disease Control and Prevention
1600 Clifton Rd.
Atlanta, GA 30333
phone: (800) 232-4636
e-mail: cdcinfo@cdc.gov • website: www.cdc.gov/ncbddd

Established in 2001, this center promotes the health of babies, children, and adults with disabilities by working to identify the causes of birth defects and developmental disabilities and to promote the health of those who live with them.

National Institute on Alcohol Abuse and Alcoholism

5635 Fishers Ln., MSC 9304
Bethesda, MD 20892-9304
phone: (301) 443-3860
website: www.niaaa.nih.gov/Pages/default.aspx

The National Institute on Alcohol Abuse and Alcoholism works to reduce alcohol-related problems by conducting and supporting research, collaborating with other organizations on alcohol-related work, and disseminating research findings.

National Institute on Disability and Rehabilitation Research

US Department of Education
400 Maryland Ave. SW, Mailstop PCP-6038
Washington, DC 20202
phone: (202) 245-7640 • fax: (202) 245-7323
website: www2.ed.gov/about/offices/list/osers/nidrr

The National Institute on Disability and Rehabilitation Research provides support for research related to improving the lives of individuals with disabilities.

National Organization on Fetal Alcohol Syndrome

1200 Eton Ct. NW, 3rd Floor
Washington, DC 20007
phone: (202) 785-4585 • fax: (202) 466-6456
e-mail: information@nofas.org • website: www.nofas.org

The primary goal of this organization is to eliminate birth defects caused by fetal alcohol exposure and to improve the quality of life for individuals and families affected by fetal alcohol disorders. The organization provides information and resources on fetal alcohol disorders for individuals, families, educators, and health-care professionals.

SAMHSA Fetal Alcohol Spectrum Disorders Center for Excellence

2101 Gaither Rd., Suite 600
Rockville, MD 20850
phone: (866) 786-7327
e-mail: patricia.getty@samhsa.hhs.gov
website: www.fasdcenter.samhsa.gov

The FASD Center for Excellence is housed within the Substance Abuse and Mental Health Services Administration (SAMHSA), part of the US Department of Health and Human Services. The center's mandates include exploring and developing systems of care for FASD prevention and treatment, and determining ways to deliver that care to individuals who need it.

For Further Research

Books

Joyce Cooper-Kahn and Laurie Dietzel, *Late, Lost, and Unprepared.* Bethesda, MD: Woodbine House, 2008.

Jody Allen Crowe, *The Fatal Link: The Connection Between School Shooters and the Brain Damage from Exposure to Alcohol.* Denver: Outskirts, 2009.

Liz Kulp, *Braided Cord: Tough Times In and Out.* Minneapolis: Better Endings New Beginnings, 2010.

Liz Kulp and Jodee Kulp, *The Best I Can Be: Living with Fetal Alcohol Syndrome or Effects.* 3rd ed. Minneapolis: Better Endings New Beginnings, 2009.

Stephen Neafcy, *The Long Way to Simple: 50 Years of Living, Laughing, and Loving with a Person with FASD.* Minneapolis: Better Endings New Beginnings, 2008.

Joanna H. Sliwowska, *Prenatal Alcohol Exposure and Its Effects on Hippocampal Anatomy and Function.* Hauppauge, NY: Nova Science, 2010.

Jennifer Poss Taylor, *Forfeiting All Sanity: A Mother's Story of Raising a Child with Fetal Alcohol Syndrome.* Mustang, OK: Tate, 2010.

Periodicals

Shane Anthony, "'No Desire to Drink Anymore.' Convicted of Involuntary Manslaughter in the Death of Her Newborn from Alcohol Poisoning, Sherri Lohnstein Has Rebuilt Her Life," *St. Louis Post-Dispatch*, September 3, 2008.

Harolyn Belcher, "Fetal Alcohol Syndrome: An Undiluted Danger," *Pediatric News*, August 1, 2008.

Pam Belluck, "Lawsuit over Adoption Raises Disclosure Issues," *New York Times*, April 28, 2010.

Danny Buckland, "Binge Mums Cause Rise in Special Needs Kids; Booze Poisons Babies in Womb," *Daily Mirror* (London), July 9, 2010.

Libby Copeland, "Drinking While Pregnant," *Toronto National Post*, October 18, 2010.

Renata D'Aliesio, "Pregnant Albertans Admit More Alcohol Use; Smoking Rates Up," *Toronto National Post*, October 12, 2010.

David Derbyshire, "Drinking in Pregnancy More Dangerous for Older Women," *Daily Mail* (London), July 21, 2010.

Julie Griffiths, "Drink Link to Childhood Troubles," *Community Care*, January 28, 2010.

Marguerite Kelly, "Fetal Alcohol Syndrome's Long-Lasting Impressions," *Washington Post*, November 27, 2009.

Janelle Miles, "Danger of Alcohol in Pregnancy Backed," *Courier-Mail* (Brisbane, Australia), October 9, 2010.

Michele Munz, "Fetal Disorder Has Lingering Effects: When a Mother Drinks in Pregnancy, Her Baby Faces Harm Long Past Childhood, Researchers Discover," *St. Louis Post-Dispatch*, October 14, 2010.

Kate Pickert, "When the Adopted Can't Adapt," *Time*, June 28, 2010.

West Australian (Perth), "Saving Babies from Alcohol. A New Research Project Is Looking at the Health and Learning Damage Caused by Mothers Drinking During Pregnancy," September 25, 2010.

Internet Sources

Ira J. Chasnoff, "How Much Alcohol Is Safe?" National Organization on Fetal Alcohol Syndrome, 2010. www.nofas.org/How_much_alcohol_is_safe.pdf.

KidsHealth, "Fetal Alcohol Syndrome," June 2008. http://kidshealth.org/parent/medical/brain/fas.html.

March of Dimes, "Drinking Alcohol During Pregnancy," November 2008. www.marchofdimes.com/pregnancy/alcohol_indepth.html.

National Center on Birth Defects and Developmental Disabilities, "Fetal Alcohol Spectrum Disorders: Alcohol Use in Pregnancy," Centers for Disease Control and Prevention, October 6, 2010. www.cdc.gov/ncbddd/fasd/alcohol-use.html.

N. Young, S. Gardner et al., "Substance-Exposed Infants: State Responses to the Problem," Substance Abuse and Mental Health Services Administration, 2009. www.ncsacw.samhsa.gov/files/Substance-Exposed-Infants.pdf.

Source Notes

Overview

1. Michael Dorris, *The Broken Cord*. New York: HarperPerennial, 1990, p. 65.
2. US Department of Health and Human Services, Substance Abuse and Mental Health Services Administration, "Fetal Alcohol Spectrum Disorders by the Numbers," FASD Center, 2007. www.fasdcenter.samhsa.gov.
3. Bonnie Buxton, *Damaged Angels: An Adoptive Mother Discovers the Tragic Toll of Alcohol in Pregnancy*. New York: Carroll & Graf, 2005, p. 201.
4. Buxton, *Damaged Angels*, p. 183.
5. Diane K. Fast and Julianne Conry, "Fetal Alcohol Spectrum Disorders and the Criminal Justice System," *Developmental Disabilities Research Reviews*, 2009, p. 256.

What Are Fetal Alcohol Disorders?

6. Francis Perry, "My Life with FASD," *Visions*, Spring 2006. www.heretohelp.bc.ca.
7. William J. Szlemko, James W. Wood, and Pamela Jumper Thurman, "Native Americans and Alcohol: Past, Present, and Future," *Journal of General Psychology*, October 2006, p. 435.

What Is the Cause of Fetal Alcohol Disorders?

8. Gabrielle Fimbres, "Born on the Bottle . . . Drunk for Life," *Tucson (AZ) Citizen*, December 1–6, 1997. www.comeover.to/FAS/Citizen.
9. The Fetal Alcohol Spectrum Disorders Study Group, "Statement on Light Drinking During Pregnancy," December 2, 2008. http://fasdsg.org.
10. Bruce Ritchie, "Birth Moms—a Personal Perspective: Economics of Beverage Alcohol," FASLink Fetal Alcohol Disorders Society, 2005. www.faslink.org.

What Are the Effects of Fetal Alcohol Disorders?

11. Sherry Martz, "Symptoms of Babies with Fetal Alcohol Syndrome: My Son's First Year," Associated Content, April 1, 2009. www.associatedcontent.com.
12. Susan Rose, "Kate's Story," *ABILITY*, January 31, 2006, p. 18. www.abilitymagazine.com.
13. Cara Hetland and Tom Robertson, "Part 3: Living with FASD as an Adult," *Fetal Alcohol Syndrome: The Invisible Disorder*, MPR News, September 7, 2007. http://minnesota.publicradio.org.

How Can Individuals with Fetal Alcohol Disorders Be Helped?

14. Jeanne, "Our FASD Stories," *Real Stories, Real Lives* (blog), Minnesota Organization on Fetal Alcohol Syndrome, 2010. www.mofas.org.
15. Anique, "Things I Want Social Workers to Know," *FASD Connections*, May 2004. www.fasdconnections.ca.

List of Illustrations

Index

Note: Boldface page numbers indicate illustrations.

About the Author

Formerly a university professor, Sandra Alters is a science, health, and education writer based in Orange, California. She has authored nearly 100 books and articles, including textbooks, reference books, and children's books.